Shannon's
Book

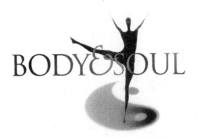

BODY&SOUL

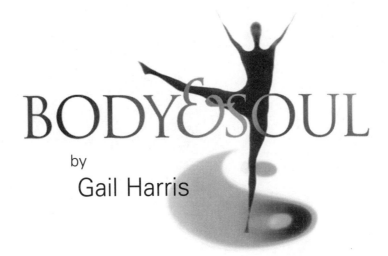

BODY & SOUL

by
Gail Harris

Kensington Books

http://www.kensingtonbooks.com

KENSINGTON BOOKS are published by

Kensington Publishing Corp.
850 Third Avenue
New York, NY 10022

Library of Congress Card Catalogue Number: 99-61846
ISBN 1-57566-481-X

First Printing: April, 1999
10 9 8 7 6 5 4 3 2 1

Printed in the United States of America

For my Dad,

Who showed me how to live

For my husband and son,

Who taught me how to love

And for all those

Who devote their lives to healing

CONTENTS

ACKNOWLEDGMENTS

In any project, large or small, the best creations are co-creations. This one, surely the largest project of my life, requires a great many thank-yous. In a list so long, I'm almost certain to have left someone out. You know who you are; please accept my apologies along with my thanks.

To the many who fed me and made me part of their families along the way—from Judy and Ed Connell in Panama City, Florida, to Ruthie and Jack Jennings in Tallahassee, to Carol and Andy Hiller in Newton, Massachusetts, and Ellen and John Shattuck of Washington, D.C.

To the late, ever-gracious Charles Kuralt, who kindly arranged a job interview for me at WBTV, the station where he got his start in North Carolina; and to the incomparable John Greene, its news director, who managed to persuade the personnel department in 1973 that even though they already had one woman reporter, it would probably be okay to add another. Both truly launched my television career.

To Ira Jackson and Michael Dukakis, who recruited me, and the admissions committee of the Kennedy School of Government at Harvard University, who accepted me: my eternal thanks for the opportunity to fill in the blanks of my formal education. Their collective faith in me transformed my life forever, even as it led to a less lucrative but far more satisfying place in public television. To my agent, Alfred Geller, who believed in me even when he didn't always agree with the wisdom of my career moves.

To Steve Atlas, David Liroff, Dan Everett, Henry Becton, and all the fine folks at WGBH-TV, where I spent four-and-a-half incredibly happy years. To Christopher Lydon, friend and co-anchor, whose writing style and analytical abilities still leave me shaking my head in awe.

To Amy Entelis, ABC News talent scout extraordinaire, whose gentle push gave me the chance of a lifetime to work as a correspondent for *Nightline*, and who understood when family obligations made it impossible for me to stay.

To Bob Gordon, Claude Pelanne, Ted O'Brien, Ellen Molle, and the rest of my colleagues at WABU-TV, who struggled and fought and bled together as we tried to accomplish the impossible—champagne public affairs programming on an apple cider budget. Still, it was an effort worth making, and I have many happy memories from my four years there.

To Ellen Hume at the PBS Democracy Project, and Andy Walworth and company at New River Media, for the opportunity to co-host the *Follow the Money* series for PBS on campaign finance reform. It should probably be illegal to have so much fun while covering such a serious topic. And to Ray Suarez, my brilliant and witty co-host, who helped make every moment a joy.

To Alan Foster at PBS, whose green light for *Body & Soul* in December of 1997 meant that a long-awaited dream was about to become reality. To David Thorne at New Age Publishing, who loved the idea from the start. To Dean Gaskill, Doug Weisman, and J. Dolan Barry, who were willing to invest their time in the project long before I could pay them. And to Bill Moyers and Ken Burns, both of whose work has long been an inspiration, for offering advice and encouragement early on.

To the talented and wildly idiosyncratic producers, editors, and others who have come together to turn the *Body & Soul* series from a good idea into even better television. To Adrienne Leicester Smith, whose inventive ideas and hard work as producer of the demo tape helped make it possible for there to even be a series, and whose subsequent programs have been as substantive as they were imaginatively produced. To Sue Yanofsky, unit manager (the most thankless job in television), who was also there from the beginning, getting us organized and keeping us on track. I will always be grateful to you both. To production assistant Michelle Chow, whose cheerfulness amid a million daily interruptions continues to amaze me. To producers Paul Stern and Drew Pearson, to Susan Bredhoff Cohen and Eric Neudel—you all do extraordinary work. Your care in crafting memorable programs made the task of creating a book that would reflect the series a challenge as well as a joy. To Avid editor Rob "Bubba" Kirwan, whose laconic manner masks a razor-sharp mind, and whose hard work is legendary. To Guy DeFeis, who moved from videography to post-production supervising and back again without missing a beat, and who managed to keep getting the programs to PBS on time. To Joel Olicker, who proved himself to be not only a fine on-line editor but a first-rate producer. To Betty Scharf, the invaluable shaper of content for both the book and television series (and keen-eyed spotter of misplaced commas and misspelled chyrons): without her thoughtful suggestions and ongoing contributions as a writer and editor, this book would still be a jumbled pile of pages on top of my desk. Her sense of humor was a bonus, as we somehow managed to keep laughing despite some fairly impossible deadlines. To Jeannet Leendertse, whose graphic design and layout skills knocked our socks off from the start, and whose ability to turn computer disks crammed with information into neat and orderly book chapters—and at lightening speed, mind you—has been truly impressive. To Beau Wright, who came to manage the website, got pressed into helping us proof and edit, and wound up making an important contribution to the chapter on mindfulness in sports. To Michelle Murray and the rest of the crew at Daniels Printing, who turned squiggles on a Zip drive into an actual book. And to Anne Palmer, our literary consultant, who guided us through the publishing jungle from concept to completion with wisdom, grace, and panache. To Robyn De Shields, Michael Shepley and Simone Bloom Nathan—I couldn't ask for a better station relations/publicity/outreach team. Your enthusiasm and expertise have been crucial to our success. To Steve Olenick and crew at Audiolink, who frequently had to drop what they were doing to accommodate one of our last-minute audio needs. To Jim Scott, who composed all the original music for Body & Soul, including its theme; each note added such depth and texture to the pictures on the screen. To everyone at the design firm of LoConte Goldman, who understood what I wanted even when I couldn't express it very well, and went on to create a series of evocative images that became the show open and logo. To Phil Gay—my director and producer in the past, and my friend, always—and his partner Jeff Northrup, designers of the *Body & Soul* Website. I am grateful to all those whose hearts and minds have been given so freely, throughout this project.

To the generous friends whose support made the television series possible: to Peter and Kay Bernon, James and Paula Gould, Grover and Starr Daniels, Charles and Nathalie De Gunzburg, to Bob Glassman and John Plukas at Wainwright Bank, to new friends Michael and Margie Baldwin and Mary Norton Shands—I appreciate you all so much. I literally couldn't have done it without you.

To my best friend, husband, and partner, Richard Abrams, who was initially puzzled when I first began to meditate every day, then became an enthusiastic proponent when he saw how much happier and calmer it made me. He has always been my biggest fan, just as I am, his. To my son, Michael, whose arrival 12 years ago brought me the greatest joy of my life and who continues to make me proud every day. To the people who are technically my in-laws but in every other way my second set of parents, Joan and Herbert Abrams. Their love and support have always been there to prop me up. I am more grateful to all my family (that includes you, Aunt Joan and Uncle Nelson!) than I will ever be able to express.

Finally, to my fellow seekers, who I hope will find help, comfort, and inspiration within these pages—my thanks to you all. You are the reason why this project was worth doing.

INTRODUCTION

Welcome to *Body & Soul*—the companion book to the PBS series on mind, body, and spirit, which began airing in January of 1999 on public television stations across the country.

It has long been my belief that television is very good at telling stories and piquing interest. What makes it frustrating is when there is so much more to say than can fit into 30 minutes on TV. Hence, this book. It features extended interviews with some of the most interesting and provocative thinkers today, and covers far more material than we could pack into each program. Knowing that the book was coming helped get us through the teeth-gnashing stage of editing, as we lamented all the "good stuff" that got left on the cutting-room floor.

This book, like the series, is intended as a "way in" for those who've heard a little about complementary therapies and want to know more, as well as an affirmation and expansion for those who have been interested in health and well-being for years. For many of us, this is an extremely exciting time, as we witness the integration of the best of Western medicine with the wisdom of ancient healing techniques.

Over the past twenty years, I have personally read and benefited from hundreds of books on these topics. No single book, including this one, can cover everything there is to be said on health, happiness, and well-being. What we have attempted is to provide an overview of the 13 most compelling issues of life at the turn of the century, from managing stress to creating better relationships. Both the series and this book offer the opportunity to hear from some of your favorite experts in a relaxed and informal setting, and introduce you to dozens of people who have benefited from what these experts have to say.

One note: I conducted all of the extended interviews and many of the "sidebar" interviews myself. For interviews conducted by a program producer, the questions are noted as coming from *Body & Soul*.

So—enjoy. Be happy, be healthy, and most of all—be well!

—*Gail Harris*

1. STAYING HEALTHY IN A STRESSFUL WORLD

Life is in the breath. He who half breathes, half lives.

Proverb

In the interests of full disclosure, you should know that in many ways this book—and the television series from which it comes—was inspired by the work of Dr. Herbert Benson, whose pioneering efforts in mind/body research 30 years ago led to the founding of the Mind/Body Medical Institute at what is now Boston's Beth Israel Deaconess Medical Center.

I first met Dr. Benson in October of 1987. I was then working as a correspondent for ABC News *Nightline* and had come to the clinic in pursuit of a story on psychoneuroimmunology—the medical name for the study of the mind/body connection. The clinic staff was obliging and helpful, and Dr. Benson was patient as he answered my questions, then submitted to the usual cutaway shots of the two of us talking. I smile now as I look back on that scene. There I was, yet another earnest and well-meaning but essentially uninformed reporter, plying him with the sort of questions that he had no doubt answered dozens of times. At the time, it was fascinating, but basically one more story in a 15-year string of (usually) interesting assignments.

One of Dr. Benson's illustrations was especially captivating, however. During a trip to Tibet, he had shot videos of Tibetan monks inside a mountain cave in temperatures of 40 degrees Fahrenheit, as they dunked sheets into water until they were sopping wet, and wrapped the sheets around their bodies.

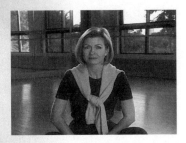

Then they went into a deep meditative state. Within a space of three to five minutes, you could see steam rising from their near-naked bodies as the *sheets began to dry*. After 35 minutes, the sheets were completely dry once again. That got my attention. As a child, I had often wondered: if we were only using 10 percent of our brains, what was the other 90 percent there for? What else might it—might we—be capable of?

As the crew and I stepped into the crisp autumn air outside the hospital, our producer approached from a nearby office, where she had just placed a call to the ABC News desk in New York. Her face was ashen. "The stock market's crashed," she reported. "The Dow dropped 500 points today." I stared at her, my interest in the intricacies of the mind's interaction with the body momentarily forgotten in the adrenaline rush of this new development. It was certainly a memorable way to fix the date of the Benson interview in my mind forever.

Eleven years later, the stock market has risen and fallen any number of times, and sharing what I've learned about health and well-being has changed from "just another story" to my life's defining passion. As I began developing this television series, the best place to start seemed to be where for me it all began—at Dr. Benson's mind/body clinic in Boston, where he and his staff still toil patiently, trying to help the rest of us learn to slow down and live.

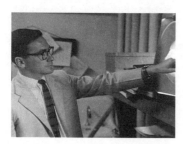
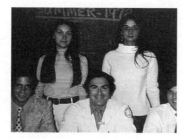

HERBERT BENSON

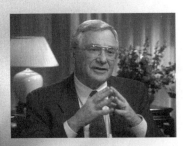

Herbert Benson, M.D., is the Chief of the Division of Behavioral Medicine and the founding President of the Mind/Body Medical Institute at the Beth Israel Deaconess Medical Center in Boston. His three decades of research into the mind/body connection has been chronicled in six books, including the seminal *The Relaxation Response* and *Timeless Healing: The Power and Biology of Belief*. He is regarded by many as the godfather of modern mind/body medicine.

HARRIS: For the benefit of those of us who haven't heard this story, how did you first begin discovering this mind/body connection 30 years ago?

BENSON: As a cardiologist, I was fascinated why some of my patients had high blood pressure in my office but didn't have high blood pressure on the outside. So I asked the question, could it be stress? In those years, it was really beyond the pale to even consider that stress, something in the mind, could affect the body. I decided to follow up on that and went back to Harvard Medical School to the Department of Physiology to see whether I could set up an animal model for stress-induced high blood pressure. We were successful. We were able to show through operant conditioning, which later became biofeedback techniques, that we could actually have the monkeys increase or decrease their blood pressure on cue.

Then some young people came to me and said, 'Why are you fooling around with monkeys? Why don't you study us? We think we can effectively control our blood pressure. We practice transcendental meditation.' I was already on the edge. Colleagues were saying to me, 'You're throwing away a very promising career with this stress mind/body approach,' so I said to these young people, 'No.' But they kept coming back, until finally, I said, 'Why not.'

These were the days before human studies committees. So in the middle of the evening, these people would come in a side door, and I would put in intravenous lines, interarterial lines, measure their out-breath, and measure their metabolism before, during, and after the practice of meditation. The changes were dramatic. By the simple act of meditation, there was decreased metabolism, that is, a decreased amount of energy the body was utilizing, a decreased rate of breathing, decreased blood pressure, different brain waves, all by the simple act of them changing their thinking.

In one of those wonderful, historical accidents, the room in which I was doing these experiments was the room in which Walter B. Cannon, who was Professor of Physiology at Harvard Medical School at the turn of the last century, had done his experiments which had defined the fight-or-flight response, or stress response, in which there was increased blood pressure, an increased heart rate, an increased rate of breathing. This looked like the opposite. I said, 'Oh my heavens, what are we looking at here?' It made no sense to me that transcendental meditation would be the only way to evoke these physiological changes, so I went back to the steps that they use in transcendental meditation. First there was the repetition of a word, a sound, a prayer, a phrase, or even a repetitive muscular activity. The second step was when other thoughts would come to mind, they would passively let them go and come back to the repetition. Using that model, I went back to the religious and secular literatures of the world to see whether or not these two steps hadn't been described before, and it was amazing. Every single culture of humankind that had a written history had these two steps within it, normally within a religious context. And ultimately, the state of deep calm and physical changes achieved by practicing the two steps we started calling the 'relaxation response.'

HARRIS: You've actually said that some 60 to 90 percent of all doctor office visits are stress-related. That seems like an incredibly high figure.

STRESS

"What is stress? Stress comes from any situation or circumstance that requires behavioral adjustment. Any change, either good or bad, is stressful."

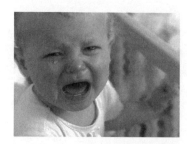

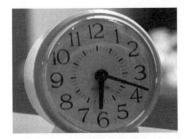 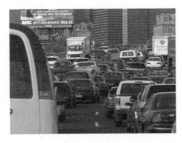 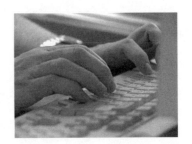

R E L A X

BENSON: First of all, what is stress? Stress comes from any situation or circumstance that requires behavioral adjustment. Any change, either good or bad, is stressful, and whether it's a positive or negative change, the physiological response is the same. There is a secretion of adrenaline, nor-adrenaline, epinephrine and nor-epinephrine. Those hormones change the mental as well as the physical components of our body. Those hormones lead to increased anxiety, increased anger and hostility, increased mild and moderate depression. They contribute to high blood pressure, hypertension, most heart disease, and angiopectorus. Even heart attacks can be influenced by these hormones. Then there are a number of gender issues directly related to these hormones. In women, PMS is made worse. Ovulation and infertility have been shown to be stress-related. Later in life, the hot flashes of menopause are both increased in frequency and severity by these hormones. In men, sexual performance and sperm count are both affected. There's insomnia; over 60 million Americans suffer from insomnia. It's costing our nation hundreds of billions of dollars.

The relationship of stress to health is compounded when we learn we have a serious disorder. Say you're told you have breast cancer. You are no longer Jane

Medication and meditation

In a recent study at the UCLA School of Medicine, 22 people with high blood pressure were taught stress reduction techniques, such as biofeedback, deep breathing, and the use of relaxation tapes. Seventy-three percent were able to keep their blood pressure under control with lower levels of medication, and over half were able to safely stop taking medication altogether. In a control group of 17 people who did not learn the relaxation methods, only a third were able to reduce their medication levels.

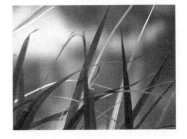

Bob Morris

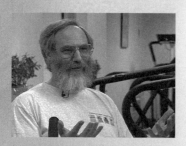

LIFE

For most of his adult life, Bob Morris would have claimed with complete sincerity that he was not a particularly stressed person. Although he had a demanding schedule of teaching and research as an academic computer scientist, he had always felt lucky to enjoy his work. So when he started waking up regularly in the middle of the night, unable to fall back to sleep, it became another opportunity to head toward his computer.

"I never thought of myself as a worrier. I saw myself as a problem-solver. If I woke up thinking about what was coming up the next day or the next week, my solution was to fix whatever it was. So I'd get up and work—and that's not a great thing to do at 3:00 a.m. because you end up wide-awake until morning. Sometimes I'd only get a few hours of sleep a night for weeks at a time."

Four years ago, at the age of 50, Bob started experiencing an uncomfortable sensation in his chest. A series of tests revealed that Bob had blocked coronary arteries, a serious heart condition. When his cardiologist suggested an angioplasty, Bob asked if he could try adopting a heart-healthy lifestyle instead. As Bob wasn't in any immediate danger, his doctor agreed. Bob is grateful to have had that option. "All surgery does is buy you time anyway. You still have to change your habits even if you have surgery. I saw hamburgers on the one hand, and life on the other—it didn't seem like a very difficult choice."

Joining a group program at the Mind/Body Medical Institute's Cardiac Wellness Program helped Bob begin to change the habits of a lifetime. He started improving his diet and incorporating regular exercise into a previously sedentary routine. But it's the relaxation techniques he's learned that have given him a new perspective on how he'd been living his life.

"I realize now I've never been very good at sudden changes in plan. The biggest stress for me was always a change from what I expected, even if there was nothing I could do about it. I didn't realize that a lot of what I saw as problem-solving behavior was really worrying or even obsessing about the past and the future. For me, the purpose of yoga is to get to meditation, and the purpose of meditation is to let go of the future and the past and really live in the present."

After completing the first phase of the program four years ago, Bob continues to attend weekly meetings as part of a graduate cardiac

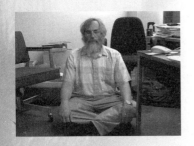

group. His medical condition shows significant improvement, and his wife, Celia, reports a marked difference in the way he handles everyday frustrations. "He's much better at realizing when the situation isn't worth getting all stressed about. He's always been tense when we're stuck in traffic. If I'm driving, I can almost feel him wanting to take over the wheel. That automatic reaction is still there, but now he's able to recognize it and let it go."

Taking control over how he responds to stress has not only left Bob a calmer person, but also one who's considerably more rested. "I still sometimes wake up in the middle of the night, but now I make an effort to stay in the present, accept whatever it is that's bothering me and move on. So I'll read a magazine or Dilbert—anything but work. I usually can't keep my eyes open for more than 10 minutes."

Smith. Suddenly, you're Jane Smith, breast cancer patient, and that adjustment of the image of who you are leads to the fight-or-flight, or stress response, which leads to these hormones. Frequently, the symptoms present early in many disorders come not from the disease itself, but from our adjustment to the disease. The 60 to 90 percent that sounds so outrageously high when you first hear it, starts to make much more sense.

HARRIS: When you also think about all the everyday things that happen that put us under stress—not just life-threatening diseases, which we can obviously understand would be stressful, but sitting in a traffic jam, waiting in a long line, being impatient for any number of reasons—it sounds as if we deal with this over and over every day without necessarily thinking that it's stress that we're experiencing.

BENSON: Exactly. Humans have always been under stress. There's always been famine, pestilence, and Huns on the horizon—interpersonal problems, male/female problems, have always been there. But what's different about modern-day life is the sheer amount of information and number of circumstances to which we have to adjust. Remember, stress comes from any situation that requires behavioral adjustment. Look at what's happened in the workplace. Traditionally, women would be at home, and men at the workplace. Now women are juggling two careers. Look at what the electronic age has done to us. Within seconds, we know of a plane going down. We know of a revolution halfway around the world. Couple that with the Internet, and the amount of information to which we now have to adjust is overwhelming. We are eliciting the fight-or-flight response repeatedly, not only with respect to health but also in our everyday lives, and this frequently leads to symptoms.

HARRIS: Who are the people who come to the Mind/Body Medical Institute? What are they looking for?

BENSON: People who come to the Mind/Body Medical Institute are those who are suffering from an ailment that has a stress component to it. It's vital when you think of the Mind/Body Medical Institute that you recognize how we approach health and well-being. It's akin to a three-legged stool being held up by one leg of pharmaceuticals and a second leg of surgery and procedures. So we use traditional medicine, with its awesome effects, on the 10 to 40 percent of people where it works. But we also add a third leg to that stool, where people can take advantage of what they can do for themselves. That third leg is self-care, where we have several components. One is the relaxation response, which is the physiological counterpart to the stress response. Nutrition, exercise, stress

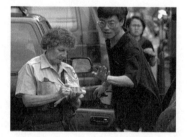

What is stress?

Human beings have an innate response, often called the fight-or-flight response, to situations of real danger. This triggers the secretion of certain hormones along with an increase in blood pressure, breathing rate, metabolism, and muscle tension to help us fight or flee a perceived threat. The problem today is that our bodies can't always distinguish between real danger and the pressures of modern life, such as juggling conflicting responsibilities, meeting deadlines, or dealing with traffic. As a result, some estimate that the stress response may occur 50 times a day in the average person. People exhibit prolonged episodic stress in a number of ways: they may become anxious, irritable, angry, withdrawn, or depressed. Over time, stress can contribute to a variety of chronic health problems, such as high blood pressure and irregular heart rhythms, which can put people at risk for heart disease. Untreated stress can also make it more difficult for people to stop certain behaviors, such as smoking or excessive drinking, or implement desired changes, such as improving eating habits and exercising regularly.

Jean Rekemeyer

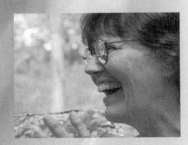

L I F E

Looking back at her life, Jean Rekemeyer can say without fear of contradiction that she's been no stranger to stress. During one six-month period, this mother of three filed for divorce, underwent major surgery, and lost a job.

Through it all, she followed the rules she had learned growing up. "I come from a family where you weren't supposed to have problems of any kind—I was supposed to be perfect. I'd always been an anxious person, but even when my knees were shaking, you'd never know it. I was taught not to wear my pain on my sleeve."

Jean's family history also included the knowledge that both of her parents had been diagnosed with heart disease, which took her father's life at the age of 57. Several years ago, Jean confronted her own heart problems when she was told her cholesterol and blood pressure levels were too high. Her doctor advised medication, but after hearing a lecture on stress management by Dr. Herbert Benson, Jean elected to participate in a cardiac wellness group at the Mind/Body Medical Institute instead.

Applying the clinic's techniques didn't come easily for Jean at first. "It took a while for me to adapt to the exercise and nutrition components of the program, but the meditation was by far the hardest part. Here I was trying to achieve this deep relaxation, and instead I would feel almost panicky because I just couldn't quiet down my mind. Then when I was able to quiet down a little, the meditation created so much anxiety that I would get asthma attacks. I had kept my feelings under wraps for so many years it was like taking a cork out of a bottle. Little by little, I began to understand how to slow down and relax."

In time, Jean was able to see the physical and emotional benefits of sticking with the program. When her blood pressure and cholesterol

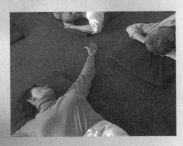
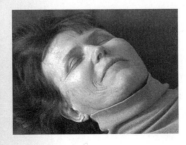
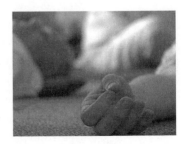

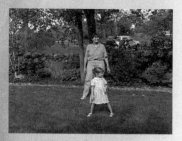 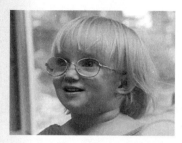 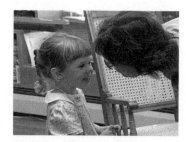

went down, she was thrilled at what she'd accomplished without medication. But Jean's greatest reward may be the dramatic change she sees in her outlook on life. "I feel like I've moved 180 degrees from where I was before. In some ways, it's like I'd always been clinging to life. I couldn't just let go and have fun. I finally understand that everything isn't my fault. I'm still a very private person, but there's a lot more laughter in my heart."

It's a change that's affected all aspects of her life, enriching her relationships with her grown children and four small grandchildren, and enhancing a successful second marriage. "I have a sense of control over my anxiety now. When I find myself in an anxiety-producing situation, I have a little routine I do. I take a deep breath, let it out, and say to myself, 'Let it go.' You know, it works."

management, and the belief system of the patient are added to that, and we integrate them in a unique fashion. It's not, today is nutrition day, or today is stress management day. Every day we deal with an entire package that we make specific to the disease we're treating.

Our results have been rather dramatic. When you add that self-care component, we can effectively reduce medicines for hypertension. We can effectively treat the symptoms of cancer, the symptoms of AIDS. We have wonderful results in terms of infertility. Dr. Alice Domar, who directs our Mind/Body Center for Women's Health and the Mind/Body Program for Infertility, is now finding up to 40 percent pregnancy rates within six months after completing our program. In our sleep disorders group, Dr. Gregg Jacobs is now having 75 percent cure rates of sleep onset of insomnia. To the extent that any disorder is caused or made worse by stress, the self-care aspect can make a tremendous difference.

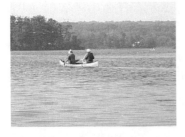 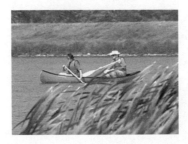 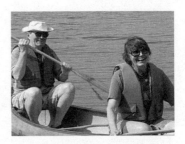

HARRIS: If such a huge number of physical problems are caused by stress, it almost sounds as if what we're saying is that if you eliminate the stress, you get rid of the physical problems.

BENSON: What we're saying is that a very large number of disorders are caused or made worse by stress. We don't want to go too far because this is a mental sort of thing; you'll get into guilt situations which are really counterproductive and erroneous. For example, there is no data whatsoever to show that stress causes cancer. There's a lot of talk about it, but there is no data to support it. However, stress could alter the course of a cancer. So, we should view all diseases as having many components. Stress might be a large component or a small component, but treat that disease first with appropriate pharmaceuticals, appropriate surgical procedures, appropriate radiation or what have you. Recognize that there are components that might be stress-related, not exclusively, but a component. Treat that as well.

HARRIS: Once having begun to integrate these self-care techniques into their lives, do most people who come to the Mind/Body Medical Institute stick with it? Do they find that their lives are transformed by it, or do they do it for a little while, and then say, 'Well, I didn't have time,' or, 'I couldn't fit it in,' or come up with some other excuse?

BENSON: At the Mind/Body Medical Institute we have sessions in the Division of Behavioral Medicine. These are groups of people who have a given disorder, and they meet for an hour to an hour and a half weekly, for roughly 10 weeks. Now at about the third week of such sessions is when people start recognizing changes. They begin saying, 'This is life transformational. I see the world differently.' That never changes. We found that in one group with hypertension, three to five years later, most still evoke the relaxation response regularly. More importantly, their attitude towards their lives has changed, which sort of cuts off stress at the front end. They say, 'Why am I getting upset about this? I can't do anything about it. Let's get on with my life.'

HARRIS : I would think it would also be helpful for people just to feel that they have some control over it, that there is something that they can do if they're feeling stressed.

BENSON : Control is a vital issue here. It's the one word that crops up over and over again in our analysis of what happens to people after our groups. What we hear is, 'I feel more in control. I'm no longer like a cork bobbing on a sea. I can control my emotions. I can control the physiological responses to my emotions, and it's wonderful.'

HARRIS : You've written about the faith factor and 'remembered wellness.' Why is remembered wellness such an important tool?

BENSON : One of the most powerful aspects of healing—the placebo effect—we have ridiculed. We say, 'It's all in your head. It's a dummy pill.' But we find that in many disorders placebos are effective 50 to 90 percent of the time—50 to 90 percent in angina pectoris, asthma, skin rashes, rheumatoid arthritis, and all forms of pain.

HARRIS : So how do you account for that?

C H O O S E

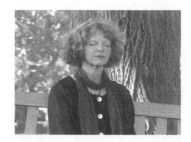

Stop, Breathe, Reflect, Choose

A major part of the program at the Mind/Body Medical Institute is learning how to manage stress. In addition to practicing the relaxation techniques of meditation, deep breathing, and visualization, participants learn how to identify their automatic emotional and physical reactions to stress, such as feeling depressed or noticing a tightness in their shoulders. Then they are taught how to break the cycle with these four steps:

- **Stop:** Don't let negative thoughts make the situation worse than it really is.
- **Breathe:** Take several deep breaths to release physical tension.
- **Reflect:** Focus your energy on the problem at hand.
- **Choose:** Now you can choose the best way to deal with the situation.

BENSON: First of all, we have to look at the components that make up the placebo effect. There are three, and they are all belief-related. First is belief on the part of the patient. Second is belief on the part of the healer or practitioner. The third component is the relationship between the two, the belief that comes from a solid relationship. Let's start with belief on the part of the patient. Japanese students were studied who were allergic to the wax of a lacquer tree leaf, like our poison ivy. They were blindfolded. One arm was stroked with lacquer tree leaves. The other arm was stroked with chestnut tree leaves to which they weren't allergic. When they were told that the lacquer tree leaves were chestnut tree leaves, there was no rash. Conversely, when they were told that the chestnut tree leaves were actually lacquer tree leaves, they did break out in the rash. That was a result of their belief and not the substance itself.

With respect to the second component, belief of the healer, let's look at angina pectoris. Angina is a constrictive heart pain brought about by a deficiency of oxygen to the heart muscle. That diagnosis has not changed in over 200 years, going back to an early English definition. But a number of therapies have come along like cobra venom, vitamin E, bizarre surgeries that shouldn't and couldn't work, but when they were believed in, they were 70 to 90 percent effective in alleviating the angina. The electrocardiogram would actually change to normal, and exercise tolerance improved. When they were subsequently disproved and doctors no longer believed in them, their effectiveness dropped to 20 to 30 percent.

The third component of the placebo effect is the belief that comes from the relationship between the healer and the patient. A study was done at

HEART

A heart to heart for women

Ask a random sampling of American women what disease they fear most and chances are the majority will answer: breast cancer. In fact, the leading cause of death for women is heart disease, claiming half a million lives each year. That's six times the number of women who die from breast cancer annually, and more than all types of cancer deaths in women combined. However, in a 1997 survey of one thousand women 25 and older conducted by the American Heart Association, only eight percent thought of heart disease as the greatest threat to their health.

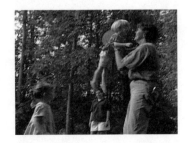

Massachusetts General Hospital where people were either seen in a cursory fashion prior to their surgery or seen compassionately by the anesthesiologist. It was double-blinded. When the code was broken, those who were seen in the more compassionate fashion required half the amount of medication, and on the average, were discharged 2.7 days sooner than the other group.

HARRIS: How can we make this work for us then? If this is such a powerful source of healing, how do you incorporate it into your life?

BENSON: The way we can take advantage of the placebo effect is, first of all, to get rid of its name. We should call it something else. What it really is, is remembered wellness. If you take a pill even though it's a sugar pill, but you believe in that pill's efficacy, you will remember what it was to be without the pain, without the rash. In other words, you can remember wellness, which is what we're calling the placebo effect, and that memory is translated into physical changes in the body.

HARRIS: How important is the choice of language here? Because remembered wellness, just on its face, sounds so much more positive than saying the placebo effect.

BENSON: Thoughts in our minds are often realities for our mind. So whether you are actually seeing it or seeing it in your mind's eye, from the brain's point of view, that's a reality. Your thoughts can have enormous power. You can actually be chased by someone or dream you're being chased, and the reaction will be the same because it's a reality in your brain. We could take advantage of that, and by appropriately believing in what can heal, we can remember those patterns in our brain and turn on remembered wellness.

HARRIS: Is that different from the faith factor, which you've also written about?

BENSON: The relaxation response is one component of the faith factor. The second is your belief system. Use the two together. In other words, first prepare your mind by quieting it, opening it up, and then use positive thoughts, remembered wellness, to bring about appropriate healing. Now, you see what makes this so fascinating is that each of us has a belief system, and we can tailor our therapies to the belief of the patient, whether it's secular, or religious. First of all, how do we do that? We give them a choice of how to evoke the relaxation response; their repetition can be secular or religious. Say you choose a secular repetition, such as the number 'one', the word

Roger Tackeff

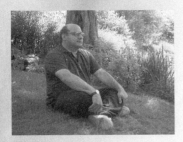

L I F E

Beneath the outwardly placid countenance of Boston real estate developer Roger Tackeff beats the heart of a passionately committed historic preservationist. At age 44, twenty years into his career, he remains deeply dedicated to saving the city's historic fabric and improving the community in which he lives. Since graduating from the Mind/Body Medical Institute program two years ago, his biggest challenge has been how to use that passion constructively instead of allowing it to eat him up.

"My problem was, I was trying to do too many things at once: be the perfect dad, perfect husband, successful professional, involved in a lot of community activities...It was all starting to drive me crazy," says Roger now. "And with a family history of heart disease and diabetes, I began worrying in my mid-30s that I was going to self-destruct if I didn't do something. I had a great need to accomplish a lot, but how do you channel those burning fires in your belly into something constructive?"

Roger still has the drive and ambition that led him through Harvard Business School and into a successful career, but now he's learned how to modulate them.

"It was fear that got me to the mind/body program. For me, there was this high pitch of stress that went on all day. I'd be late for a meeting with four urgent phone calls that had to be returned and two people in my office who had to see me before I left. And then I'd be worried about getting everything done to get home in time for dinner, because it's important to be there for dinner with the family, and I could just feel the stress level building and building. I could literally feel myself clenching up inside."

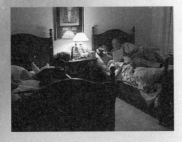
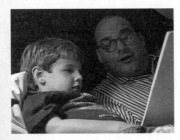
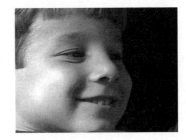

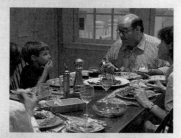

The first advice Roger received at the Mind/Body Medical Institute was to stop worrying about an extra 40 pounds he had spent a life-time trying to lose.

"I walked in and said, 'Okay, tell me how to lose weight'. They said, 'Don't go on a diet, change your lifestyle. Add exercise to your life. Use the relaxation techniques we're going to teach you. Learn to use food appropriately. You can start by only eating when you're hun-gry.'" Roger laughs at the memory. "Now, you have to understand: I wouldn't know what the sensation of hunger is. I've been eating for the wrong reasons since the day I was born. But now I do eat differ-ently. And I walk three miles every day at 5:00 a.m. Not because I want to, necessarily, but because I feel so much better when I do."

At first, Roger says, he felt out of place in the mind/body program. Almost everyone else was at least 20 years older than he was. Many had already experienced heart attacks or had other serious medical conditions.

"I got to the program the first day, and I didn't feel like I had the right to be there. I wasn't sick enough," he recalls. "Cleverly, they teamed me up with someone who had just had a major heart attack. He was about my age, and by the way he too had a young child, a newborn baby. And he said, 'You're so lucky to be in the program now, before you have a problem. Do you know what it's like to go to sleep each night and be afraid to close your eyes, because you don't know if you're going to get up in the morning?' That took my breath away. It gave me a legitimate reason to feel that I'm doing something not only for me but something for my family as well. I'm learning how to take care of myself."

Sleep had been another issue for Roger. "I used to wake up in the middle of the night and worry. Now if I wake up, I meditate and get myself back to sleep. During the day, I use the relaxation response, sometimes more than once a day. It's not a big event; sometimes it can be short. But it makes a big difference in how I look at the world and how I let it affect me.

"I used to think that everything was a crisis. Now I understand that there are only a few things that are really important in life."

'peace', or the word 'love'. If your belief system is religious, it would depend on your religious background. You might use a prayer from that background. If you're of secular belief, believe in the medications, the proven medications. Believe in the importance of relationship. Believe in a spirituality that's nature-based. If you're of religious background, believe in God's ability to heal you. With 95 percent of Americans believing in God, that can be a very powerful healing force.

HARRIS: This sounds like such a different approach from viewing your body which you take to the doctor like you take your car to the auto mechanic. 'Here it is. It's broken. Fix it.'

BENSON: We should really have these approaches built in from the beginning of our life. To that extent, we at the Mind/Body Medical Institute have brought forth our educational programs. We are now teaching stress management and the relaxation response to young people in school, from kindergarten right on through graduate schools, and the results are wonderful. Teaching them the relaxation response in schools, early in their lives, is helping them with better grade point averages, increased self-esteem, fewer unexplained absences, and better work habits. The children love it.

HARRIS: Does meditation or the relaxation response offer kind of a key to remembered wellness and to the faith factor? Is that the way that you can begin to get your body accustomed to maybe dealing with itself in a different way?

BENSON: The relaxation response is fundamental. First of all, it counteracts the harmful effects of stress, but secondly, immediately after you elicit the relaxation response, your mind is more open. More information gets in. It's quieter. There's less static. So the way to change your thinking of things is to

AWARE

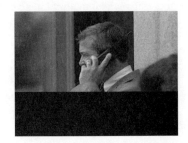

"What I've learned is that many patients are just not aware of the stress they're experiencing. After so many years of being under stress, they almost desensitize to the effect it has on them, emotionally and physically."

Aggie Casey, RN, MS, Clinical Director, Cardiac Wellness Program, Mind/Body Medical Institute

PROTECT

evoke the relaxation response and immediately afterwards to expose yourself to the kind of information you wish to get in. It could be stress management. It could be how to treat a particular disease, or it could be just changing your attitude.

HARRIS: Dr. Benson, you've written that humans are 'wired for God,' as you put it. How so?

BENSON: Our brains remember certain things, and those memories are wirings. They are highly complex nerve connections. Memories are such connections, but as humans, we are also wired for certain basic aspects of survival, some of which are innate, some of which are learned. We're wired for fear of heights, and we're also wired to learn to walk, to learn to talk, to learn to control our bowels, and to put thoughts together. Now, we are the most intelligent species on Earth. We are the only species that knows, for example, that we're going to die and know of it early. From childhood, we know that death is part of things. That's not good for us from an evolutionary point of view. Why go on? Why have children? I'm only going to die. Why put them through the suf-

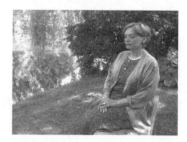

How to achieve the "relaxation response"

The relaxation response is a state of deep calm that results in a decrease in breathing, blood pressure, metabolism, and muscle tension. That state can be achieved by practicing two basic principles of meditation:

• repetition of a sound, phrase, or motion
• passively disregarding your thoughts

You can meditate sitting on the floor or in a chair, or lying down, and while walking, jogging, swimming, gardening or doing yoga. What's important is focusing your mind on the repetition of a sound or movement, and letting your thoughts go by without judgement. Studies have shown that practicing this simple form of meditation for at least 10 minutes each day can help many people protect against or alleviate anxiety and depression, headaches, heart rhythm disturbances, high blood pressure, PMS, and insomnia.

fering? The moment I'm born is the moment I'm going to start passing away. It's fascinating that every single culture of humans that has ever written, going back thousands of years, has believed in something more, that there is something after we pass away, that there's another world, and that there are powers, forces, energies out there with which we can communicate. Just as we're wired for certain fears and certain learning capabilities, so it appears we are also wired to believe in something more. We are wired for God, and that's good for us.

HARRIS: You've also written that faith is good for us. Does that mean then that we can use faith to counteract some of the stresses that we feel every day?

BENSON: I use the word faith as if it were belief. Believe in what you know to be important to you, and that belief can definitely counteract the harmful effects of stress. Believe in what you're doing to counteract the stress. Believe in relationships, and if you're of a religious nature, believe in the protective aspects of God. That's good for us because it gives us hope, and that hope is a very wonderful way to cope with many of the stresses of everyday life. Now, I'm not saying that we should all believe in God. I'm saying if your belief system is to incorporate God, and religiosity, and that kind of spirituality, that's wonderful. If you're not religious, then use another belief in which you have faith, and that belief can also help you counteract the harmful effects of stress.

HARRIS: If you were to write a prescription for good health, with all the stresses and strains people experience every day, what would that prescription be?

BENSON: The prescription for good health would be: use the drugs, use the surgeries appropriately, but build in self-care and recognize that it's scientifically based. For that, you should learn to recognize stress for what it is. You should evoke the relaxation response regularly, using a secular or religious technique depending upon your own belief system. Use appropriate nutrition and appropriate exercise. In addition, rely heavily on what you believe in. Use your own belief system and build that in as you would the pharmaceuticals, the surgery, and the relaxation response, and bring them all together. It's not that difficult.

Meditation is not an evasion. It is a serene encounter with reality.

Thicht Nhat Hanh, Zen Master

2 AGING WELL: MEMORY AND MOVEMENT

It surely isn't news that we live in a culture obsessed by youth. Anyone who has the slightest doubt need only pick up the latest fashion magazine to observe the progression of what appear to be sultry-eyed 12-year-olds, whose stick-thin bodies act as human hangers for all that expensive clothing. Not a lot of folks with gray hair in *those* pages.

As a member of that demographic bulge known as the baby boom, and as someone who has had to be concerned about how she looked on camera since age 20, I have to confess that I look in the mirror about as much as anybody. Yes, I do take note of the wrinkles that weren't there yesterday, but I began to feel better about them once I realized that most were laugh lines, and laughing—a lot!—is one of my favorite things in life. I also hope that as my fellow boomers and I march through our 40s and 50s and beyond, that together we will give new meaning to the word, "aging."

Funny, isn't it, how most of us try to push away the fact that time is passing, and that, yes, we're getting older. Yet most of us are glad to acknowledge that with our years, we've acquired experience. Wisdom, even, at least on our good days. I wonder how attitudes might change if, instead of saying, "I'm getting old," we said instead, "I have a great deal of experience. I know something about a great many things." Hmm. Puts a somewhat different face on things, doesn't it?

If we can come to terms with the fact that getting older can bring with it many positive aspects—especially as long as we are able to remain active and healthy—what is it about old age, exactly, that scares us so?

As I began mulling that one over with the *Body & Soul* producers, who range in age from 20-something to 60-something, we realized that apart from issues of general health, it's the thought of losing our memory that seems especially distressing for most of us. Now, even my 12-year-old son will wander into a room from time to time and then forget why he's there or what he came to get, so we can't chalk up each and every lapse to advancing age. Still, there is great interest and some exciting work going on in the field of memory loss, and we wanted to check it out for you.

The other perceived downside of getting older has to be how we literally move through life, how much strength and flexibility we're able to retain. Research is beginning to tell us that it's possible to stay strong and mobile, even into very old age. And the ancient Chinese practice of Tai Chi—also known as meditation in motion—can help us remain connected to the beauty and wonder of our physical bodies, no matter how many years we've had them.

So read on for some good advice on staying active and healthy from Dr. Andrew Weil and some exciting ideas about memory loss from Dr. Dharma Singh Khalsa. That commercial a few years back may not have told the whole story when it reassured us that we're not getting older, we're getting better. But getting older on our own terms is certainly possible.

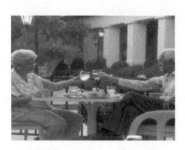

ANDREW WEIL

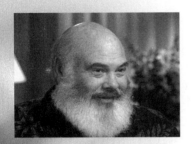

In 1971, three years after obtaining his degree from Harvard Medical School, Andrew Weil embarked on a four-year journey through North and South America and Africa, collecting information on drug use, medicinal plants and methods of treating disease in other cultures. His exploration of alternative medicine, mind/body interactions and medical botany became a lifelong focus. Dr. Weil is currently Director of the Program in Integrative Medicine and a Clinical Professor of Internal Medicine, at the College of Medicine of the University of Arizona. He is the author of seven books, including the international bestsellers *Spontaneous Healing* and *8 Weeks to Optimum Health.*

HARRIS: We've been told that the greatest risk factor for developing memory loss is age. I wonder if you think that memory loss can be treated effectively.

WEIL: First of all, I would say that memory loss, like many other functions that we look at, may not be a necessary correlate of aging. I think what we do see is that in many old people, there is somewhat of a loss of recent memory. Many people today are very frightened about more serious memory loss, especially the dementia of Alzheimer's disease. But, in fact, the percentage of older people that have Alzheimer's disease is still a small minority. As you get older and older, the percentage increases. It may be that what we call the ordinary memory loss that's accepted as normal with aging, is preventable and highly treatable.

HARRIS: How so?

WEIL: I think primarily by exercising the mind. In my view, the secret of memory is attention. If you're not paying attention when something goes past, it doesn't get filed. And the secret of attention is motivation. If you don't care whether you retain something or not, then you're not going to pay attention. It won't get filed. So I think there are a lot of things people can do to train their memories. And it may be that what we call the normal memory loss of aging is, in fact, an example of the principle of 'use it or lose it.'

HARRIS: What's your take on hormone replacement therapy as part of this?

WEIL: There is evidence, I would say not conclusive yet, that estrogen may be protective against Alzheimer's disease, and it may be that these new designer estrogens that are coming out will maximize that effect. There's also some evidence that non-steroidal anti-inflammatory drugs have a protective effect against Alzheimer's disease. There are new generations of those drugs coming out that may be much safer, that will maximize that particular effect. Those are two possibilities of things that we now have, although they may not be in perfect form, that might be both preventive and therapeutic.

HARRIS: I want to talk a little bit about the value of memory. From a very practical standpoint, obviously, it's important to remember where you left your glasses. It's also important to remember your granddaughter's name and when her birthday is. But, in a very real sense, memory is the repository of who we are. I'm wondering, if we were able to deal better with memory loss issues, whether that might not help overcome some of the fears that people have about getting older in general.

WEIL: I think that the fear of loss of memory, and the loss of identity and independence associated with that, are probably right up there at the top of the list of fears that people have about aging. There is a tremendous amount of denial of aging in our culture, and it's interesting to think about why that is. Some of it might have to do with denial of death. But I suspect that a lot of it may have to do with fears of particular kinds of losses, and very central to that, is the fear of loss of memory.

HARRIS: Do you think it's possible to grow older and still be as vigorously healthy as you were when you were young?

WEIL: I think that one secret of successful aging is to adapt to the changes that happen in the body as you grow old. There certainly are changes that happen. There's loss of elasticity, for example. There's a decline of healing ability. But those changes are not necessarily inconsistent with being in good health. There are many examples of people who grow old and reach what we call the old, old stage of life, and then have a fairly rapid decline and death without

Dharma Singh Khalsa

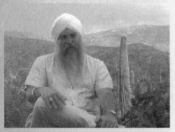

Dharma Singh Khalsa, M.D., is the founding director of the Acupuncture, Stress Medicine and Chronic Pain Program at the Maricopa Medical Center in Phoenix. He is a conventionally trained American- born physician with an unconventional appearance and way of life. As a practicing Sikh, he wears a white turban and follows a holistic lifestyle that includes meditation, yoga, and vegetarian living. His approach to treating memory loss is equally unconventional.

"In my experience," observes Dr. Khalsa, "when someone goes to a conventional doctor reporting memory loss, the doctor usually tells them that it's old age and nothing can be done about it. And if they're not old and they have a more subtle memory problem, they're told, 'Don't worry about it, because it's not Alzheimer's disease.' But if it's bothering the person, it is important.

"In addition, while it used to be thought that age-associated memory loss was a benign disorder and nothing to worry about, it's just part of aging, now it's known that patients with age-associated memory loss can in fact progress to develop the real thing, Alzheimer's disease."

For the past five years, Dr. Khalsa has been the president and medical director of the Alzheimer's Prevention Foundation in Tucson, a complementary medical program researching the prevention and reversal of memory loss. He is also the author of *Brain Longevity: The Breakthrough Medical Program that Improves Your Mind and Memory.*

"The more conservative medical camp has been looking for one factor, one pathology, and the one magic bullet that's going to affect, for instance, Alzheimer's. In the integrative medicine approach to memory impairment, we're looking at the whole brain cell and trying to impact everything. We're looking at ways to increase blood flow, energy, oxygenation; we're looking to regenerate the cell membrane.

"The greatest risk factor for developing memory loss is age, and there's nothing that anybody can do about that. As we age, the risk increases. For those 85 and older, there's a 50 percent chance of developing memory loss. Other risk factors include family history and certain types of genetics. However, there are also risk factors that we can influence, such as stress, poor diet, and lack of exercise."

In Dr. Khalsa's view, it is possible, in many cases, to prevent memory loss or reverse its progression, by applying certain techniques of

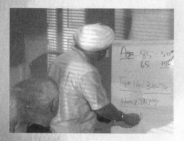 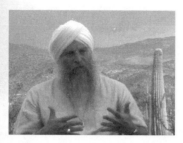 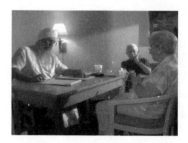

mind/body medicine that benefit more than just the brain. "The first principle of brain longevity is that the brain is flesh and blood like the rest of the body. In fact, what works for the heart, works for the head, with some variation. That's very important. The latest research shows that people who have a higher-fat diet and consume more calories are more prone to develop many chronic diseases, such as heart disease, cancer, and now, Alzheimer's disease. In addition, countries with the highest intake of fat and calories have the highest incidence of Alzheimer's.

"Stress is a key risk factor for memory loss. Cortisol is a hormone released in response to chronic unbalanced stress that acts like battery acid in the memory center of the brain, destroying brain cells over time. When we lay down initial or short-term memory, this involves the hippocampus or the memory center, which is very sensitive to cortisol. But it's been shown that even the most simple, basic relaxation or meditation technique will lower cortisol and improve many areas of mental functioning.

"Whatever we can do to lower these risks can decrease the possiblity of developing memory loss. So in the art of integrative medicine, using nutrition, stress management, and exercise—things that patients can do for themselves—can really help prevent or reduce memory loss."

In certain cases, Dr. Khalsa will recommend taking specific anti-aging drugs and hormones as the last piece of an overall program of self-care. "Hormone replacement therapy is an exciting area of research. The work on estrogen has shown that it helps to, if not prevent the incidence of Alzheimer's in women, at least to slow its development.

"Secondly, every patient that I've ever seen with memory loss has a low level of the hormone, DHEA. It's a very mild male hormone, and as it goes down from its peak at age 30 to around age 80, what happens is degenerative diseases go up, whether it's heart disease, arthritis, cancer, or memory loss. So it's believed by anti-aging physicians that if we replace DHEA levels to a point of where it is at about age 30, we can in fact reverse some of these findings."

But Dr. Khalsa cautions against unsupervised use of some newly available substances. "With anything you do in medicine, there's a risk/benefit ratio. For instance, with DHEA, there's a very real concern because it affects a man's prostate gland. What really bothers me the most is that anybody can go into a health food store and start taking DHEA. I think that's the greatest controversy, because it's extremely important to monitor the patient's blood levels and the function of the prostate.

"People get excited when I talk about the drugs and the hormones. I tell them, 'This is not a magic bullet. The drugs and hormones make up only about 10 percent of the program. I want you to exercise first, I want you to improve your diet, take the supplements and learn to do the meditation techniques in the mind/body exercises. Then only in certain advanced conditions, we'll talk about the drugs and hormones.' Taking care of your brain is possible, but it's the total program that works."

suffering, without disability. I think that's a goal that more of us could work toward. And I think there are specific actions that we can take in the way of adjusting lifestyle to increase the chances that we're going to be in that category.

HARRIS: Let's be a little more specific about those changes.

WEIL: Of the studies on aging that have been done, one factor that stands out greatly is the importance of exercise. Physical activity seems to be an across-the-board panacea that increases people's chances of arriving at old age in a better rather than a worse condition. That doesn't necessarily mean a strenuous workout every few days. It might mean just increasing general life activity, rather than sitting around and being a couch potato.

HARRIS: What about something like Tai Chi, which is very gentle. It's not vigorous.

WEIL: That might serve the purpose quite well. Keeping the body moving, that's a big one. In the mental/emotional/spiritual realm, the one that jumps out is engagement—engagement with the world, engagement with society, engagement with other people. That seems to be highly protective in old age.

So those are just two specific areas, physical exercise and engagement, that look highly protective and seem to increase our chances of arriving at old, old age in better shape.

HARRIS: I want to ask you about gingko biloba, something that a lot of people are very interested in. In *Spontaneous Healing*, you quoted from a letter from someone who raved about it, who said it had done everything from help the hearing loss in his 94-year-old mother to curing his own depression. You also noted that this is the sort of thing that most doctors and scientists would kind of drop into the trash can as being anecdotal evidence. Why do you think anecdotal evidence like that needs to be listened to?

WEIL: Science begins with raw observation. You look out, you notice something in the world that strikes your attention. You see it again. You form a hypothesis and test the hypothesis. That's how we extend our knowledge. The first step is raw observation, and in medicine that means paying attention to individual case examples. If you discard that first step, if all of that goes into the wastebasket labeled anecdotal evidence, you lose your source of hypotheses. That's where we get ideas. The ideas should then be tested, but the ideas come from experience and observation.

HARRIS: So you're not saying just blindly follow the anecdotal evidence. You're saying use that as a starting point.

WEIL: Use it as a starting point. That's what gives you the ideas to do your experiments.

HARRIS: Because isn't the other side of it that if you use anecdotal evidence as is, what's great for one person might be terrible for another?

WEIL: Absolutely. This could be a special case, or the effect you observe may have nothing to do with the cause that you say is the cause. That's why you have to test it. But if you have a good intuitive sense in medicine, and you see interesting case examples, you can get a pretty good idea of what things are likely to pan out, and to design experiments that are likely to be productive.

HARRIS: You've also noted that the placebo effect can be a tremendous therapeutic ally for doctors, certainly in dealing with disease. Is that also true of aging?

WEIL: Absolutely. In fact, I would go further than that. I think the placebo effect is the meat of medicine. This is what medicine is all about. You're trying

Sydne Bortel

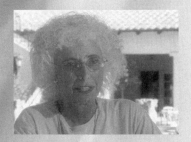

LIFE

About seven years ago, when Sydne Bortel was in her early 50s, she began noticing subtle changes in her ability to remember.

"Much of it was just the routine, where are my glasses; where are my keys. I've lost my car in the parking lot. Much of what I was feeling I could accept as normal middle-aged stuff. But there were some specific things that really upset me. When I was speaking to a group, I wouldn't be able to recall certain words. I would find myself always searching for simpler words to say the same thing."

Sydne was married, the mother of two grown children, and had a challenging job as the clinical director of a family service agency. As time went on, Sydne found her memory lapses increasingly disturbing. "When I would be writing something, a note, I would forget letters in a word. When I was writing a check, I might literally forget what year it was.

"For years, whenever I mentioned any of this stuff to anyone, I was reassured, 'Oh, it's normal, it's nothing. Everybody has this happen.' I didn't believe it. I knew some of it was normal—I certainly knew that it was worse when I was under stress or had to perform. But the change had been so great for me, I began to worry about it a lot."

Sydne's worries about her memory were compounded by a family history of both parents having been diagnosed with Alzheimer's.

"One of the real shockers was one day when I was putting my car in the garage, I forgot that I had a garage door opener. I got out of the car and I started to put the key in the garage lock. Those were some of the things that said this is different, this is not normal."

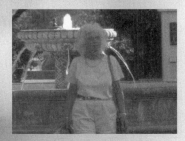

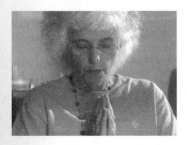

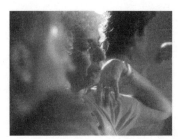

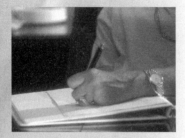

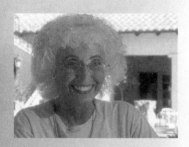

When Sydne expressed her concerns to her internist, he suggested that she have some testing done to allay her fears. Several years ago, Sydne underwent a complete battery of tests.

"There were some signs that were of concern to me and the tester, but his attitude was very much the same as any other medical professional that I talked to during this time: 'You don't have any dementia yet; there's nothing to do about it. Watch it, and get tested again.' Generally the response was kind of a placating 'Wait until it gets bad, and then maybe there will be a pill for it.' There was no suggestion of anything that I could do to turn it around or prevent it from getting worse."

One day, Sydne came across Dr. Dharma Singh Khalsa's book on what he calls "brain longevity." Although she had never heard of his work before, she was intrigued enough to investigate.

"I'm a very skeptical person, so reading all this stuff about nutritional supplements just made me say, 'Come on now,' because I've always felt people who pop a lot of vitamin pills and such are very impressionable, and that was never me. I was taking a little bit of ginkgo, my multiple vitamins, my calcium, but that was about it.

"But I decided if someone is offering you some hope, it might be a good idea to try it. I went very carefully over the chapters about nutritional supplements and began to make lists of Dr. Khalsa's recommendations. Little by little, I got myself out to the health food store and started buying these supplements. The numbers of pills I have been taking per day are the biggest pain in the neck. I counted my pills the other day, and I think I was taking 26 pills a day.

"I worked with this nutritional program probably for about three or four months, and I didn't see much change at all. But in the last couple of months I have begun to notice some differences. And on some levels it's very subtle, and on other levels it's quite remarkable.

"It's as if the cobwebs are clearing. When I read something, I know what I've read. My speech is clearer; I don't lose words or mispronounce them the way I did before. When I write, I'm not leaving out letters.

"I think there is much less stress on me now. I feel freer. I'm not worried about myself. And it's not only worry—it's all the effort that goes into covering up, not letting anybody see. Now I'm not thinking about how will they feel if they think I'm losing my memory or getting Alzheimer's. I'm just much more relaxed in the world."

to find out how to stimulate healing responses in people. If you can do that with less and less direct intervention, which is likely to be toxic, you're practicing better medicine. You want to get the maximal healing response with the least intervention. In terms of geriatric medicine, I think there's enormous room for that. I even reviewed some literature recently about tests of new drugs for Alzheimer's disease, which is pretty dismal. We haven't come up with many things. But one of the clear findings was that just being enrolled in a study on Alzheimer's disease produced measurable improvement in the things we look for in people suffering from Alzheimer's disease. That's a placebo response, whether you attribute it to the engagement of being in a program or the possibility of getting better.

HARRIS: It has to make you wonder if some of the issues we encounter as we age is because we expect our bodies to fall apart.

WEIL: Absolutely. And in a way this is the model our society in particular creates. I just saw an article in the Sunday *New York Times* about a group of senior citizens who were on an elder hostel trip, not the usual kind, to a remote area in Alaska to be with an Inuit community. This was dramatic not only because these older people were going on a much more rigorous kind of trip than they normally would, but they would also be visiting a society which had a very different value placed on age. The Inuit elders were the most valued members of the community. They were valued for their experience, and they were treasured. That's certainly not the model that we create in this culture. The ageism of our society is expressed in many different ways, but I think there is a common cultural belief here that old people are likely to be trouble: getting in the way, unable to take care of themselves, unproductive. That's the kind of model we have, so it's not surprising that many people manifest that reality.

HEALING

"You're trying to find out how to stimulate healing responses in people. If you can do that with less and less direct intervention, which is likely to be toxic, you're practicing better medicine. You want to get the maximal healing response with the least intervention. And in terms of geriatric medicine I think there's enormous room for that."

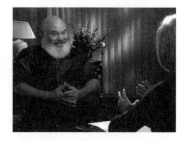

HARRIS : It's kind of a chicken and egg problem. If we felt more positive about getting older, then perhaps people would believe that they could be vigorous.

WEIL : I think that's a big part of it.

HARRIS : How can we feel more positive about aging?

WEIL : I think through education and also by looking at examples of people who show a different model for aging. The optimistic research that's been done suggests that many of the deficits of aging, whether it's muscle weakness, inactivity or depression, are reversible. If people are given training or support, they can rather quickly bring a lot of this function back.

HARRIS : Strength training, for example.

WEIL : That's a dramatic one, and it's very well documented.

HARRIS : What about the role of nutrition in aging? We all pretty much know what it is we're supposed to eat. But what about some of the more exotic things?

WEIL : One of the problems of looking at aging research is that it's very important to distinguish the diseases of aging from the process of aging. Much of what we see that we say is a consequence of aging may actually be the consequence of diseases that people become more susceptible to when they get older. That susceptibility may have to do more with lifestyle than with aging itself, in particular with nutrition, with activity and so forth.

One category of nutrients that I'm very interested in are the essential fatty acids. There is a great deal of literature about the role of the central fatty acids in brain function. One particular central fatty acid called DHA that's in fish

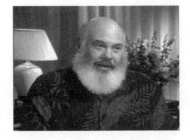

"It's very important to distinguish the diseases of aging from the process of aging. Much of what we see that we say is a consequence of aging may actually be the consequence of diseases that people become more susceptible to when they get older. That susceptibility may have to do more with lifestyle than with aging itself."

oils and walnuts and flax is generally deficient in the American diet. This is the principal constituent of cell membranes in the central nervous system. It's very possible that, if your diet over your lifetime is deficient in this, the architecture of the brain could be weak, and leave you susceptible to degenerative brain diseases. That's a very practical piece of information. People should be aggressively supplementing their diet with salmon, herring, sardines, flaxseeds or walnuts, and other sources of these hard-to-get fatty acids.

HARRIS: And yet that kind of information isn't generally known.

WEIL: One reason for that is that we're still not teaching medical students nutrition, or at least practical nutrition. My great concern is how we're going to change medical education to produce a new generation of physicians that know not only about nutrition but lifestyle in general, body/mind interactions and so forth.

HARRIS: Which brings me to the question, is aging well difficult? If you've had a lifetime of bad habits, but decide that you want to change your life, that's not always so easy.

WEIL: It's not always easy. But I think it's very important to note that research shows that at whatever point you begin to make those changes, you get benefits quickly. An example of that is smoking cessation. People may have smoked all their lives, and yet from the moment they stop, there begins to be improvement in lung function, in cardiovascular function and so forth. It may take awhile to catch up to people who haven't smoked, but the effects start right away. I think the conclusion from that is, it's never too late.

Tai Chi: A matter of balance

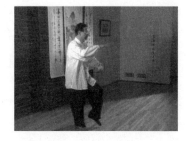

According to a 1997 research study at Emory University in Atlanta, practicing the ancient Chinese martial art of Tai Chi has been shown to reduce the risk of falls in the elderly by 48 percent. Falls among the elderly pose a serious health risk that can lead to disability or even death. Fear of falling keeps many other seniors inactive. With the proper instruction, this gentle system of deliberate movements can make a significant difference in helping older people improve their sense of balance.

HARRIS: What about some of the other things, particularly in terms of physical exercise, for somebody who views the golden years as the time that they just want to kick back and take it easy. What do you say to them?

WEIL: What you say to them is that exercise doesn't need to be strenuous, but that moderate, regular physical activity causes an increase in a sense of well-being, decreases aches and pains, increases flexibility, offers great protection against the possibility of falling, and if you do fall, protects against the possibility of sustaining a fracture. That evidence is overwhelming, and I believe that if you give people accurate information, a lot of them are going to be motivated to make the necessary changes.

HARRIS: What about age-related stress? For many people it can be an extremely stressful time. There's fear about the future. There's anxiety about everything from finances to health. Are there ways of alleviating stress specifically for people who are aging?

WEIL: I don't know that there are any ways that are different from people of other ages. I think that people of all ages need to deal with stress and neutralize its effects. The particular techniques that I teach a lot are breathing exercises, because they're so simple, they take very little time and no equipment, and everybody can do them. There are very simple breathing techniques that are great for relieving stress. I think another thing is try to work on the sources of stress. For example, a major source of stress in older people is that they've retired, and their occupation may have provided them with many sources of satisfaction, including engagement with other people. So one wants to look for a way to replace that. Where are you going to get that kind of support, if you're not getting it from your job?

HARRIS: Where do you?

WEIL: I think you have to work to create that in your own life, if you realize that's something important that you need.

HARRIS: There are a lot of people in situations where they're concerned about aging parents. They might want to suggest, 'Well, Mom, I think Tai Chi would be a wonderful thing for you to take up.' Is it appropriate to try to encourage that?

WEIL: Absolutely, although I think you need to explore with people what is consistent with their belief system and their own habits. Tai Chi may not be

Martha Moline

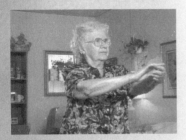

LIFE

Martha Moline may be 88 years old, but that's not how she defines herself. "I don't even think about my age. I think that's because I'm exuberant; I enjoy life. I love doing things and traveling."

A fall in 1981 which seriously injured her left knee slowed Martha down a little, but it didn't stop her. She kept on walking with the help of a cane. In 1994, Martha fell again and broke the same leg. After a long course of physical therapy, she graduated from a walker back to a cane. When Martha was given the chance last year to participate in a Tai Chi program designed specifically for older people, she embraced the idea with her natural enthusiasm.

"When they told us they thought we would all be a great deal better for this particular exercise, I was ecstatic. 'Oh my, don't tell me I will be able to walk without my cane again.'"

Although the Tai Chi movements seemed strange at first, Martha began to look forward to the twice-weekly classes led by Tai Chi grand master Xan Shu. "For instance, this movement we do with our hands coming up like this and then coming back down, where we're really concentrating, it does something for your whole body. It seems to give you balance and a sense of grace. It's not a sort of old-ladyish type movement."

Over time, Martha has seen a significant improvement in her mobility and sense of balance. "My knee still gives me some problems, but there is such a difference in how I can move it. I associate this with all of this 'oiling of the joints,' all of these motions that we do. My body feels stronger and this leg feels really strong again. In fact, I'm able to walk up stairs.

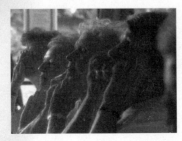 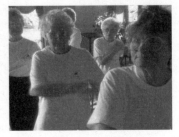

"My sense of balance is better, too. Balance, to me, is not falling to one side, the way I have been in the last few years because of my impairment—and being able to turn, the simple motion of turning, picking up something, being able to come back up and feel as though I'm not going to fall.

"I think overall it's very helpful because you learn to concentrate, and by concentrating you can throw some worries aside. It just sort of gives you a glow when you get through with these classes.

"I would say if you have the opportunity to take Tai Chi lessons, by all means, do it. It doesn't make any difference if you're old, young, or middle-aged. I think it's just wonderful for your body and your soul."

appropriate for some people, but aqua aerobics in a swimming pool, in a class, might be just the right thing, or some kind of organized walks with other people. It takes some work to figure out what's the appropriate activity to suggest.

HARRIS: Any guidelines?

WEIL: I think it's very individual. You present a menu of options and facilitate making it happen. Another problem that we experience in this culture is that old people are very segregated. It would be great if we had new kinds of communities in which there was a range of ages, where old people could be more integrated into the life of the community. That would be moving a little bit toward that Inuit goal.

HARRIS: Grandparents working with kindergarteners.

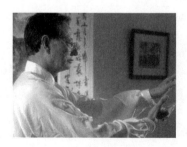

CONNECTIONS

WEIL: Exactly.

HARRIS: I'm wondering if you can paint a picture for us of what a great old age could be and how you get there.

WEIL: To me, a great old age would be getting to enjoy the rewards of having lived long, that is, to be valued for your experience, for surviving, to be honored, to remain highly engaged with the world and other people, to continue to do work that's productive. A lot of work that older people do now, such as taking care of young people, is not paid, and is not considered productive work. But it certainly is productive. We need to change our view of that. A great old age also means remaining physically active and independent in all of the basic functions of life, and that when you near death that decline is relatively quick, without an extended period of suffering, of disability and lack of independence.

How memory works

Our brains are designed to handle two kinds of memory. Short-term memory is the "working" memory, which allows us to use information in the present moment without necessarily keeping a record of it. For example, short-term memory is how we might remember an unfamiliar phone number long enough to dial it. Long-term memory is created when experiences are retained in the area of the brain known as the cerebral cortex. The cortex responds to stimulation by forming connections within its thicket of 10 billion nerve cells. If a new connection is activated over time, the neural network will become even more developed. The result is a lasting memory. Information which has emotional significance, or is related to things we already know, is much more likely to remain in the memory bank. Random associations are remembered far less often.

Alzheimer's is a particular disease of the brain, which initally robs individuals of their short-term memory. Unlike other memory disorders, the condition progresses to also affect the capacity to think or reason. It's been said that a person with Alzheimer's doesn't just forget his keys; he forgets what his keys are for. Estimated to afflict 10 percent of the population over 65, Alzheimer's is a complicated syndrome which requires expert medical diagnosis.

People of similar ages, whether young or old, show great variety in their capacity to remember. While getting older may slow some of us down mentally or make us less precise, age by itself will not necessarily result in memory loss.

HARRIS: Is it fair to say that you absolutely believe that it is possible to age well? That aging and disease and illness and feebleness don't have to go together?

WEIL: I think they don't have to go together. It is possible to work on preventing and treating and correcting the common illnesses that we see increase in frequency with age, up to a point, obviously. But I think that a great deal of what we now see as disability and disease associated with aging is actually separable from the aging process itself, and can be approached with changes in lifestyle.

HARRIS: If you were to write a prescription for good health as one gets older, what would be on the pad?

WEIL: Certainly attention to a good diet that was preventive of cardiovascular disease, of cancer and so forth. Judicious use of supplements that could increase physical resistance, immune function, healing ability, brain function. Stress protection measures and having some techniques at your disposal to deal with stress. Physical activity of the sort that we've discussed that would maintain the body in good condition and be a preventive against the kinds of disasters that happen to old people. Mental practice to keep the mind sharp and to keep memory from diminishing. And the kind of social engagement that I've talked about.

3 CREATING WELLNESS: TAKING TIME, MAKING TIME

I suspect that I made a friend forever when I asked producer Drew Pearson to check out the Omega Institute for Holistic Studies in upstate New York. Since its creation more than 20 years ago, Omega's mission has been to "bring spirituality into daily life." It is one of the original places to go for a contemplative retreat, or a workshop on anything from Tai Chi to yoga to Nigerian drumming.

Drew did seem to be the perfect person to send. He is an accomplished documentary producer and photographer, the sort of person who can blend into the woodwork long enough to observe and record important moments without intruding on them.

So when he came into my office one day with the Omega catalogue open to Stephan Rechtschaffen's week-long workshop on wellness, I agreed right away that it was worth a visit. After all, we both felt, wellness is more than the absence of disease; it is an attitude, a way of appreciating and fully experiencing every moment of your life. If these folks at Omega could teach us, and we could pass along to you some ideas on how to do that in just one week, so much the better.

I still have the memo Drew faxed to the office upon his return home to Maine. "When you get in your car to leave Omega after six days of concentrated work within the geography of its campus," he wrote, "there's an initial sense of disorientation. Can I still drive? You haven't turned on an engine for that whole time, or seen television, or listened to the radio, or read a newspaper. Arriving at the first rest stop on the Massachusetts Turnpike, there is

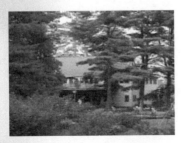

the outside world, big-time: stacks of newspapers, noisy cars, crowds of people wolfing down burgers…"

After you come behind the scenes at Omega with us, I hope you'll take away the same feeling of peacefulness that he did. And if you can remember in the coming weeks to slow down for a moment to savor life, all of our hard work will have been worth it.

STEPHAN RECHTSCHAFFEN

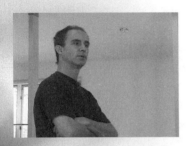

Stephan Rechtschaffen, M.D., is the president and co-founder of the Omega Institute in Rhinebeck, New York. He has organized symposia and educational programs across the country, and lectures on wellness, nutrition, and longevity. Dr. Rechtschaffen is the author of *Timeshifting: Creating More Time to Enjoy Your Life.*

HARRIS: I want to talk about a concept that you've described as timeshifting. I think many people would read that as, 'Oh good, I'm going to have more time in my life—by driving my car, having my breakfast, talking on the phone and listening to the radio, all at the same time.' But that's not what you're talking about, is it?

RECHTSCHAFFEN: Timeshifting is really different from time management. Time management is where we're going to fit in as many things as we can, and get the treadmill of life going faster. The problem is that nobody creates more time. Timeshifting is about having a different quality of time. It's not doing everything at once. It's experiencing what we're doing, and being here while we're doing it.

HARRIS: But what does that mean, really? What does it mean to be living life 'fully in the now,' as you put it?

RECHTSCHAFFEN: Timeshifting is like riding a 20-speed bicycle. When you go up a steep hill, down an incline, on the flat or around a curve, you shift gears. Time, to me, is simply the rhythmic dimension of life. Each moment has a different speed to it. Sometimes we're bored and we think things are so slow. Other times we're excited and it's going very fast. Life has a way of shifting its rhythms. But what happens is we get stuck in one gear too much of the time, and in modern society, it's usually fast-forward. Timeshifting is about learning how to slow down when something is happening in our life that requires our attention in different ways: spending time with our child; spending time with loved ones; spending time smelling the flowers of life.

HARRIS: So you're not really talking about living life in slow motion.

RECHTSCHAFFEN: Absolutely not. And that's why I don't call it down-shifting. I love to be able to go really fast. I love to do sports that are fast. But what happens is, we get addicted to just going fast. I met a gentleman, a very successful entrepreneur, on his way to climb a mountain. He was telling me that the only thing that turned him on anymore were death sports—helicopter ski-ing, bungee jumping, hang-gliding—things that always put him at high levels of risk. When we go at full speed all the time, we look for these thrills, instead of realizing that what we have in regular life is very full. We just have to slow down to appreciate it. It's like there's an area you always drive by very quickly, and one day you decide to walk. All of a sudden, you're asking, 'When did they build this house? When did this tree grow here? When did these flowers bloom?' If we slow down, we get a different appreciation of life. But nowadays, you have to learn to cultivate that ability.

HARRIS: So much of life seems to be coming at us so much faster than it used to. There was a time when you would get a letter in the mail. Now we get it by fax or e-mail, and we feel as if we have to respond immediately. How do you build in slowing down when everything is coming at you so quickly?

RECHTSCHAFFEN: You learn that when the fax comes in and you have to respond, you do it quickly. But what I look for is those moments in between. You're waiting for an elevator, and it isn't coming. You're impatient, you're thinking, 'When is that elevator going to come?'—as though doing this will make the elevator come. You can tell this internal rhythm when you see somebody tapping a pencil on the table, or their foot going up and down, waiting for something to happen. Those are the moments we can learn to simply breathe.

I focus on the breath a lot, because the breath is the one physiological func-tion—the only one—we need all the time. You can't live without breathing. So whether we're conscious or unconscious, we continue to breathe. But when we're stressed, our breathing is short, shallow, rapid. When we're able to take a breath and slow down, we're able to relax the whole system. In a moment, you can go from a fast breath to a relaxed breath, so the breath is an excellent way to slow down. What I do, if I'm waiting for that elevator and I feel stressed,

I'm late—I'll just close my eyes, I'll take a few breaths, and all of a sudden, there's a sense of relaxation. In modern life we're always waiting. We're stuck in traffic jams. We're waiting for doctors. There's the bank line or waiting for food. I just try and take those opportunities to breathe.

HARRIS: No matter what we're doing, I think most people feel as if they absolutely do not have enough time in their lives.

RECHTSCHAFFEN: We're always complaining. I ask people, 'Do you have enough time in your life?' And inevitably people feel that they don't have enough time. They feel time-poor. There's a sense of time sickness. It's a real epidemic in modern life. We tend to blame this feeling on external stresses. Our environment causes us to be busy. It's caring for children. It's caring for elderly parents. It's our work schedule. It's our social obligations. The truth is, we all have the capacity to change that. It doesn't take much time to be present. As far as I'm concerned, the way we create time in our lives is not by adding six hours to the day—we would just fill that, too. It's very simple. Wasting time, as far as I'm concerned, is not being here. Creating time is simply being present for this moment right now.

Too many of us have a deal about the moment. It goes like this: 'I'll be here if it feels good. And if it doesn't, then I don't want to be here.' So we spend a lot of our time avoiding being present. The problem is, all of our stress is related to not being present. Because in this moment there is no stress; it's fine. We're anxious about what's about to happen. We're remorseful about what has happened. We're regretful. 'If only I had...' But here we are, and this moment is just fine. It doesn't mean, don't plan. It doesn't mean, don't think about the future. But it allows us to go with the flow of life a little more easily, instead of always feeling like we're up against it, even on a busy schedule. I know people who have

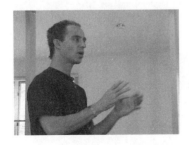
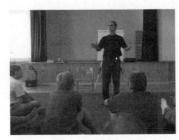
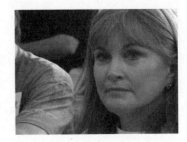

very, very busy schedules, and yet in the midst of it, they do things with serenity and with equanimity. They just take life as it comes. This is something no
one has taught us. It's something we need to be learning more, and I use
timeshifting as a way to do that. It's just shifting the rhythms to simply be here,
and take a breath when you can.

HARRIS: How did you figure this out?

RECHTSCHAFFEN: I figured this out because I found myself desperate for
time. I found myself having grown up achievement-oriented, as so many of us
are in this society, and doing one project and then another. And before I knew
it, I had three jobs. For many of us, when we don't have enough time, we see
crises develop—a bankruptcy, a divorce, a serious illness, problems with the
children, a car crash, all sorts of things. And that crisis brings us into the present moment. There's nothing like a divorce to make you be present. There's
nothing like bankruptcy to make you say, 'Oh my God, what's going on?'

Too many of us are living our lives without being aware of what's going on.
There's a bumper sticker, that says, 'Having a good time. Wish I were here.' For
too many of us, life is just passing by. We watch the children—they've gone;
they've grown up. We didn't even notice it happen. When will we get to spend
time? When we finish the project. When the kids get out of school. We're not
allowing ourselves to really enjoy our lives. And then we blame it on our environment, instead of realizing it's really us who needs to change.

HARRIS: You are a physician by profession. What does that kind of stress,
that kind of adrenaline high, which so many people live on every day of their
lives, do to us physically?

RECHTSCHAFFEN: With this adrenaline high, the adrenal gland, which is
the stress gland of the body, is continually pumping. It's why we take in caffeine, for instance. We consume large amounts of caffeine in part to speed us
up. And the adrenaline rush it gives us makes us very present, very attentive. But
then we get totally addicted to it, and we only feel okay when life is going at
this ultimate fast speed—in order for us to feel high, in order for us to feel
alive. At least 80 percent of our time is spent doing the mundane tasks of
everyday life: walking the dog, doing the dishes, the shopping, the laundry. Too
many of us look at those tasks, and we want to fast-forward ourselves through
it. We want to get on to the important stuff or the exciting stuff, and so we
miss most of life.

Rob Oberndorf

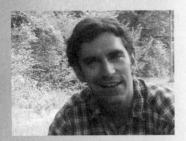

L I F E

When 32-year-old Rob Oberndorf told friends that he was planning to spend a week's vacation at the Omega Institute for Holistic Studies, the common reaction was, "You're doing what?" But no one was more surprised than Rob himself, a busy young lawyer whose vacation choices tended to run more toward adventuring in the great outdoors than venturing inward on a spiritual journey.

"I had absolutely no idea I was going to come to the Omega Institute. I planned on taking a vacation; I was burned out, and I needed the change of scenery. My original plan was to do a mountain bike camping trip out in California or Idaho, but one trip was cancelled and another ended up being sold out.

"Then a friend of mine gave me a copy of the Omega Institute catalogue. I took it, and I looked at it, and I thought, 'Yeah, right, sure, this is something I would never do.' But after the two camping trips fell through, I picked up the catalogue, and I opened up on the section of the Wellness Week program. I thought to myself, this could actually be interesting. This might be exactly what I'm looking for right now, because at this point in my life I'm trying to get back in touch with my spiritual side—something which over the last few years I've completely lost touch with.

"That spiritual side goes back to when I was in college. I had a sense then that if I had a loving heart and mind, and I could express that to others in the way I treated everyone, then that could be almost a contagious aspect which would flow from person to person to person. Then sometime after I graduated from law school and started working, I lost touch with that side of myself.

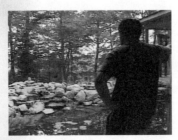

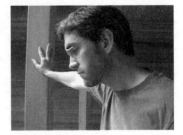

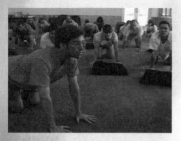

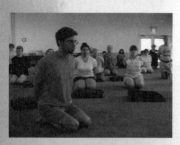

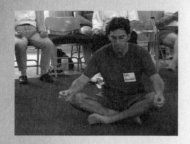

"I was good at my work, and I was considered very successful. But suddenly I was thinking to myself, well, now what? I had all these questions, but not really any sort of grounding on which to answer the questions. Finally, I realized I better sit down and take stock of who I am and what's important to me. And if I can figure that out, then I'll be able to answer the other questions."

Despite the need he felt to find some answers, Rob still wasn't sure he'd made the right choice after booking his reservation at Omega. "I'm driving out here, filled with a certain amount of apprehension, thinking: 'What am I getting myself into? Am I going to have a miserable week? Am I going to be sitting here all week long going, oh, this is so stupid?'"

His doubts turned out to be short-lived. "After the first day I suddenly realized, wow, this is great, I'm really enjoying this. I really like the people here, and what I'm learning is extremely interesting. For one thing, I've never done meditation ever in my life. I never thought I could sit still for it. But I found that as I was meditating, I could get a better sense of the things that were bothering me in my life, and how it is I want to live my life and project myself to others.

"One morning, at about 6:30, I couldn't sleep anymore. I got up and went to the sanctuary, and there was this Sri Lankan Buddhist monk, who led us through a Buddhist love meditation. First you focus on love of self, love of family and close friends, love of neighbors and those that you work with, then love of all humans in the world, and love of every living creature on the earth. And that was very, very powerful. It struck a lot of emotions in me.

"All of a sudden I was having this feeling that I don't think I'd had since I was in college. I felt this sense of freedom; this sense of being completely at ease with myself. At ease with who I am; at ease with what I believe in; at ease with how I'm interacting with other people. And I left that meditation session feeling so energized and so happy and so aware of everything that was around me.

"I knew before I came that I had lost something. I just didn't know what it was. I'm turning back inwards and exploring myself, and becoming more in tune with exactly who I am and what's important to me, and how I want to live my life. I've rediscovered that side of myself I used to be so in touch with. That's something that I can go home with, that will carry me on."

I work a lot with people about honoring the mundane, because I find the mundane part of life is a great place to practice being present and relaxed. For example, I like to do the dishes. That doesn't mean that I can't wait to do your dishes or that I want to do everybody's dishes. But in terms of my own dishes, I feel it's one thing I know I can get done, and I know I can do it right. There aren't that many things in my day that have both of those qualities. If we can be content with some of the simplicity in our life, then we start to open up life a little more.

HARRIS: It also occurs to me that if you really are paying attention to doing the dishes, then that list that goes on in your head of all the things you have to do, isn't going to be there.

RECHTSCHAFFEN: Absolutely. And that's really critical. Because if we can give ourselves some time which is a rest from all of that chatter, all of that incessant mind stuff, boy, it feels good. And what ends up happening is the answers I'm looking for emerge more easily. All of sudden I've got the answer. It's not by asking and asking, 'What should I do?' That doesn't give us the answer. It's really just by quieting down sometimes.

HARRIS: You talked before about being achievement-oriented. Do you find that some people think that success or money can, in a sense, 'buy' time?

RECHTSCHAFFEN: We have a sense that if we had more money, or more success, then we would create time. It doesn't work that way. We create time now, and then we create a life for ourselves that seems more content, more happy. It's remarkable to me that in our culture we have more goods, more services, more products than any people who have ever lived on the planet, and yet we live with a certain amount of discontent and dissatisfaction—a sort of hunger. We're like hungry ghosts in the way we live. I look at the way our ancestors lived who had much less than us, but were often more content. I think we have to find a way to balance ourselves. Otherwise, we're just going to keep thinking, 'If I only go faster, then I'll get it. If only I had more, then I'd be happy.' Yet the more I see people getting, it doesn't seem to be doing it. There needs to be a different pace. And timeshifting is about changing the pace.

Most of us live with a strange equation called 'time is money.' We start to value our time related to how much money we're making for the time. If we're doing the dishes, we think, 'Well, I could also be talking on the telephone and watching the news.' We start to be very good at multi-tasking, and trying to juggle more and more balls. This just adds to the stress load we have.

There's an opportunity here, in the everyday part of life, to really experience the simple joys of life. Now I'm not suggesting that's how we should we spend all of our time. But if we're in continual resistance to washing the dishes, or when we're washing the dishes, we're thinking about dessert, the problem is, when we get to dessert, we're not thinking about dessert. We're thinking about the movies. Everything is just slightly ahead of us, so we're never here. We always feel a little out of breath, a little stressed, just trying to get to the next thing. Even when we enjoy things, we're in the habit of thinking: 'When is the next thing happening?'

One of the things I've learned is that it's really possible to change that, and it's in changing that, that we start to regain our lives. We don't create time by going faster. We create time by simply allowing ourselves to be here. Then, what I've seen in the people I work with, and in my own life, is that all of a sudden—time opens up. It doesn't mean that I'm necessarily doing less. I still find that I'm doing a lot. But when I'm doing it, I'm not worried about what the next thing is.

HARRIS: So when you're holding the baby, you're holding the baby. And when you're doing the dishes, you're sort of feeling the water and watching the suds.

RECHTSCHAFFEN: That's right. It's very practical. It's not something esoteric. In my medical practice, when I would put people on programs oriented to wellness—exercise programs and stress reduction programs—I would see people become terrified. 'I don't have enough time now. And you're telling me to do this and this and this?' I'm not suggesting that, because I don't want to add more stress. Instead, I'm suggesting that we look at how can we start to relax a little bit in daily life. When I'm really busy, just be here for it. I'll be busy for a period of time. When I'm in crisis, that's what I'm doing. I'm paying attention to that.

CREATE

"We don't create time by going faster. We create time by just simply allowing ourselves to be here. Then, what I've seen in the people I work with and in my own life, is that all of a sudden—time opens up. It doesn't mean that I'm necessarily doing less. I still find that I'm doing a lot. But when I'm doing it, I'm not worried about what the next thing is."

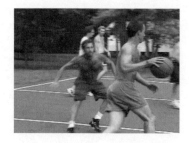

I ask people, 'What does it feel like to sit on a couch with nothing to do?' It's remarkable to hear people say they never do that, or they talk about their guilt or their anxiety. We are the most productive people who have ever lived on the planet, yet the moment we stop and just sit there for two or three minutes, we feel guilty, like we should be doing something else. It's really unhealthy for us, and I think it's fundamental to all the stress-related diseases we have. I consider time the major cause of stress in modern life. And that stress is what leads to the chronic degenerative diseases, the heart attacks, the cancers, the strokes—all of these issues that we as a society are increasingly suffering from. If we want to turn that around, we need to start paying attention to creating balance in our life.

Timeshifting is really about creating balance in everyday life. You learn how to go fast when you need to go fast. But when you don't want to go fast, you slow down. We want to learn to pace ourselves, because life is a long distance and a long time. If we want to live life well, we don't run it at the speed of a 100-yard dash the entire time. That's why people die of heart disease. They die of heart attacks before they get to the finish line, because they're going at a pace that doesn't really sustain health.

HARRIS: If you think about it, 100 years ago people lived at the pace of nature. You think about how slowly seasons change. We certainly don't live at the pace of nature, do we?

RECHTSCHAFFEN: No, we don't. It's one of the things that I emphasize—that we need to get in touch with nature again in that way. Because the world around us is about computers and the beepers that are going off. All of that is fine in and of itself. A favorite quote of mine from the author Rene Daumal goes something like: A knife is neither right or wrong, but he who holds it by the blade is surely in error. I think that's the way we are with our

P A C E

"Timeshifting is really about creating balance in everyday life. You learn how to go fast when you need to go fast. But when you don't want to go fast, you slow down. We want to learn to pace ourselves, because life is a long distance, and a long time. If we want to live life well, we don't run it at the speed of a 100-yard dash the entire time."

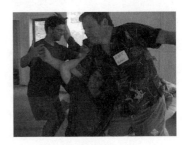

technology. It offers us wonderful advantages, but if we're always going at that speed, then we lose touch with nature. We lose touch with the rhythms of our own life. We have evolved over millennia to the bird song and the wind in the trees, and too many of us are cut off from that now. We're going at a very rapid-fire rate that is very distressing to most of us.

HARRIS: You've written about mental time and emotional time. What's the difference?

RECHTSCHAFFEN: I think the difference is in the rhythm and the rate. With mental time, our thoughts go very quickly from image to image, but feeling or emotional time goes much slower. A feeling may rise up very quickly, but the processing takes a period of time. If we get irritable with our spouse, if we get frustrated with something at work or we get upset with something that happens with the kids, instead of processing the feelings, we feel we don't have enough time, so we suppress the feelings. We consider it efficient to stay in our minds all the time. Now, that's okay. But the moment we stop, these feelings come up again. And we're not comfortable with them, so what we do is we run from them. Many of the people I work with don't stop long enough to really experience what their feelings are. We blame not having time on being so busy, but the truth is that we've created our busyness to avoid our feelings. Until we're able to allow the feelings that naturally come up in life to be processed, we end up creating busyness as an avoidance mechanism. We now have a society that's quite expert at creating busyness to avoid the real issues of life.

HARRIS: When you begin using various techniques to slow down a little bit, to build on those pauses you find in the course of your day, what happens to the flow of your day? Does it get easier? Or do you feel as if you have some catching up to do, because you're not able to do as much during the course of that time?

RECHTSCHAFFEN: As time gets faster, the moment gets shorter and shorter. When you start to find a few moments here and a few moments there to allow yourself to be present, relax, and take a few breaths, instead of being in a negative feedback cycle about time, you're shifted into a positive one. The remarkable thing is, you get more effective. When we expand the moment, we become much more effective and successful at what we do. People who really know how to be successful in their lives learn how to open the moment at the right time. We look at a great sports star like Michael Jordan with just a few seconds left in a game. But during that time, time seems to expand. Instead of thinking, 'Oh my God, am I going to get the ball in? Are we going to lose?' he's just fully in that moment. When we get stressed, we start to worry about this, and get anxious about that, and then what happens is we're not performing at our best. I find that as we start to use these techniques, the wonderful thing is not only do we create time, we become more successful at what we're doing.

HARRIS: Let me ask you about solitude. Why is solitude important in creating time for yourself?

RECHTSCHAFFEN: Many of us don't have much solitude. We have time when we're alone. We might be alone working, or doing certain chores, or shopping. But not the kind of time when nothing is going on, and we can reflect on what's happening in our lives. I know in my life I've often made decisions because somebody asks, 'What do you want to do?' and I have a quick response. Solitude allows me to slow things down so that I'm not just reacting with my mind, I'm also reacting with my gut feeling.

Too many of us fear solitude. Feelings might come up that are unresolved—we might feel abandoned, or alone, or guilty. But I believe that we only experience real serenity in life when we can sit alone and feel comfortable—sit alone and be just exactly who we are, not needing anything to change, not needing to produce anything. We become identified with being a doctor, an author, a father; all of the different ways that I show up in the world. But stripped of that, who are we? In solitude, we find out. Initially that can be terrifying to people. But until we start to spend a little more time in solitude, we never get to really see that part of ourselves, and without that we're not truly content. We're always sort of hiding, and running away from who we are.

HARRIS: It takes some confidence to do that, doesn't it, because many people would describe it as being very selfish. Is there such a thing as creative selfishness?

"Too many of us fear solitude. Feelings might come up that are unresolved; we might feel abandoned, or alone, or guilty. But I believe that we only experience real serenity in life when we can sit alone and feel comfortable—sit alone and be just exactly who we are, not needing anything to change, not needing to produce anything."

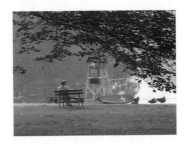

SOLITUDE

RECHTSCHAFFEN: Yes, I think there is. Unfortunately, when we prioritize time, we put work first. We put spouse and family second. Third is the everyday, mundane chores. Fourth is social responsibilities, and bottom on the list is us. But if you don't have any time, nothing gets to the bottom. Most people I see are running on empty batteries. The recharging of the battery comes from taking some time for oneself, and not necessarily like a hermit in solitude. It can be in the form of play or exercise. It can be fun. Many of us need to be nourishing ourselves more, but we have this fear that we're going to be perceived as selfish. It does take a certain amount of confidence or courage. But I think we have a lot more to give each other if we're a little more nourished within ourselves.

HARRIS. You talk about how important it is to be physical. Why does that contribute to our overall good health?

RECHTSCHAFFEN: When I play basketball there's nowhere else I want to be. I'm not thinking about the future or the past. I'm fully present. I'm like a child at play. We see the delight of our children when they're just playing. I think we need more of that. We can talk about the biochemistry, and endorphins, and about all those positive things that happen. Ultimately, I think we know it's good for us, because there's a feeling afterwards of just feeling wonderful about life.

HARRIS: What do you mean by 'creating time boundaries'?

RECHTSCHAFFEN: Most of us are so focused on productivity and achievement, but it's really important to have a certain amount of time where we're simply present and doing whatever, where we take 20 or 30 minutes and there's nothing coming out at the other end of it. This is what I call time with boundaries. We can be tinkering, puttering around the house, working in the garden, or taking a walk. We can be sitting and just listening to music. Too many of us only listen to music as background while we're doing chores. So time with boundaries is an opportunity for us to not have anything else going on but whatever we feel drawn to do at that moment. It creates a space for us to be in our own rhythm. Instead of always being called to go at somebody else's speed, we start to feel comfortable in our own rhythm. Then we find that the rest of the day proceeds at a more leisurely pace, or a pace that's more in sync with us.

HARRIS: You also talk about 'creating spontaneous time' which sounds like an absolute contradiction in terms. If you're creating it, how can it be spontaneous?

RECHTSCHAFFEN: I find the spontaneous aspect of life is sometimes where our greatest joys are. You wake up that morning and you have no idea what you're going to do. It's like a snow day, where life just opens up to us. It's like children. They're ready for whatever comes up. I think too many of us have become adults, and as adults we have everything planned. It's fine to have plans, but I know that some of the best experiences in my life have come when my plans have fallen through. So I give myself that time. I find it opens you up to a much broader experience of life, which gives us a richer feeling, and ultimately, a much healthier approach to life.

HARRIS: What about 'creating time retreats'?

RECHTSCHAFFEN: We need times where our hopes, our heart, and our spirit have a new way of experiencing life. Too many of us are closed in. We are prisoners of time, and we need to be let go. We need to break out and be a little more free. Time retreats give us an opportunity to look at our lives very carefully and decide what changes we want to make. So we say, 'Maybe when I get back, instead of always doing this, I'll do it this way.'

HARRIS: You're not just talking about creating more time. You're really talking about being fully alive.

RECHTSCHAFFEN: That's absolutely right. Because I equate time with a sense of what the soul is. In Papua, New Guinea, they have no words for hour, minute, or second. But in our language, we not only have hour, minute and second, we have nanoseconds. It's very difficult in these nanoseconds to have much of an experience of life. To experience life we need to widen what we call a moment. Instead of feeling rushed, we need to slow it down a little bit. When we shift that rhythm, we start to have a different experience of aliveness. A balance in life is to be able to go fast, and when things slow down, to go, 'This is nice.' Appreciating the full spectrum of life, that's what we're talking about.

BALANCE

"To experience life we need to widen what we call a moment. Instead of feeling rushed, we need to slow it down a little bit. When we shift that rhythm, we start to have a different experience of aliveness. A balance in life is to be able to go fast, and when things slow down, to go, 'This is nice.' Appreciating the full spectrum of life, that's what we're talking about."

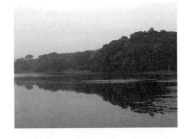

4 LENNY'S STORY PART 1
CANCER AND THE QUALITY OF LIFE

It's difficult to imagine anyone whose life hasn't been touched by cancer in some way, whether it's a friend who's been diagnosed, or a family member, or perhaps even you, yourself. Ten years ago, I watched my father die of colon cancer, feeling his anguish as the strong and vigorous body that had always served him so well seemed suddenly to become the enemy.

Cancer is a disease about which millions of words and hundreds of books have been written in the ongoing attempt to explain and understand what it is—how it progresses and how sometimes it goes away, the effect it has on those who are diagnosed with it and what it does to those who love them.

These next two chapters are not intended as either the definitive word on cancer, or on the wide range of complementary therapies that are increasingly being called upon to treat it. They are simply one man's journey through what he calls the "new normal" of life with cancer. His name is Lenny Zakim.

On his office wall in Boston you will find pictures of Lenny with presidents and priests, with prime ministers, senators and sports heroes. As regional director of the Anti-Defamation League of B'nai B'rith, his lifelong mission has been a fight for human rights and against bigotry, for harmony and against hatred, for peace and justice from South Boston to South Africa. Those who know him and many who only know of him are stopped short by the terrible irony of someone like Lenny having to take on the additional burden of an incurable cancer. They marvel—as did we, during the months we spent with him—at how he keeps on keeping on, four years after his initial diagnosis. And

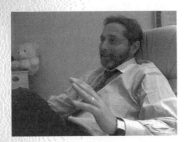

then they look at his family—his wife Joyce, son Josh, and twin daughters Shari and Deena, and they begin to understand why each moment, each breath, is so precious to him.

We were both inspired and informed by Lenny's story. We hope you will be, too.

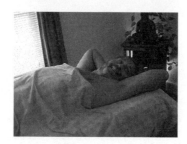

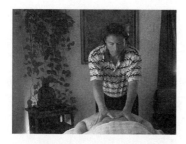

LENNY

"You can be a player. You don't have to merely wait for your own demise."

LENNY ZAKIM

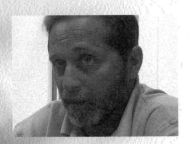

Lenny Zakim turned 45 in November of 1998. It was a birthday he wasn't sure he'd be around to celebrate, after he was diagnosed with multiple myeloma—a malignancy of the bone marrow—in January of 1995. Since that time, he has endured round after round of conventional treatments for cancer, including high-dose chemotherapy, full-body radiation, and a harrowing stem cell transplant to help restore his immune system—all treatments that he believes have helped save his life so far. It is the complementary therapies he has incorporated into his battle with cancer, however, that have changed the quality of his days, and given him a new mission: to make these therapies readily available to *any* patient who wants them. We sat down with Lenny in September of 1998 and began rolling tape. No questions were necessary, after the first one. We simply listened as he told his story.

LENNY ZAKIM: I had a really good life. And the diagnosis of cancer was the end of that life as I knew it. Being told you have cancer is still, I think, one of the three worst words you can hear in your entire life.

I remember so vividly, the room just started to spin. I became totally claustrophobic. Even though I had a couple of months of bad tests that led me to the diagnosis, I wasn't surprised, but I was devastated. You're cut out of this world that you had. It's as if Gulliver reached in. You're a Lilliputian. He pulled you out and kind of just threw you into the air. And you're falling without this parachute, or you fell down this elevator shaft and there's no elevator.

I was on automatic pilot. I didn't have a chance to process it all. It was kind of like, this isn't really happening. It wasn't denial in the true sense. It was just like

'No. I'm going to wake up and it's going to be gone.' I was always a firm believer that with single-minded determination and the energy I had, I could do anything. I was a person who slept four hours a night. Five hours on the weekend, maybe. I felt you could do anything by just working at it.

So, anyway, those first couple of weeks were really difficult. I had a meeting in Worcester about some anti-Semitic incident and on the way back I started getting really bad chest pains. I couldn't breathe. I felt like I'd eaten a couple of Thanksgiving turkeys. I pulled over to the side of the road. I really thought I was having a heart attack, and I got very, very scared. Then I drove back and I stopped at the Wellness Community in Newton, and fortuitously, they were doing a group meditation. And I went into the group. There were four of us. I had learned how to meditate when I was in college. I'd done it all through college, all through law school, and into the first years of marriage until my twins were born. Then I couldn't get away with coming home from work and going off to meditate for 20 minutes. It was too much. We had three kids under the age of three and it just wasn't going to work. I had kind of given it up and used it only in extraordinary circumstances, like before a big speech or something that I knew would be highly stressful.

So I went to this group meditation and I started to feel a little better. I started doing it twice a day, which is recommended, twice a day for 20 minutes. And within two days all those symptoms were gone. I didn't go to a psychiatrist; I didn't take any drugs. I recovered myself, my physical self, from those stress things by meditation.

I was blessed to have a very strong family and a group of friends who were with me all the time, but still, for those first eight months after diagnosis, I just did the thing. I went in for test results, and I had some pains. In June of that year, I started to have symptoms of the cancer, and I began to enter the world of true loss of control, which is what happens when you take drugs of this sort.

My doctor put me on something called Decadron, which is a very strong steroid, and I developed very, very bad symptoms: fever, severe bone pain. Just terrible pain—terrible, excruciating pain. But then it began to have some positive effects. Everything is a balance in this game, so you balance the positive with the liability of it. Then I went to Israel in July and I really began to feel the pain. At first I thought it was altitude and flying or whatever, but it was the cancer. There were times in Israel that it really was very painful, and I came back and went to see Ken Anderson [Lenny's oncologist at the Dana-Farber Cancer Institute] and he said, 'Okay, we need to accelerate.' Because they really thought I'd have a couple of years [to live].

I mean, myeloma is a very strange disease. It's very rare. Less than three percent of people in America have it, and an overwhelming percentage of people who have it are African-American—many people joked that I was taking the Black/Jewish dialogue stuff I do a little bit too seriously. A lot of elderly people get it, and that's why the fatality rates are so high, because elderly people don't have as much endurance and strength to get through it.

I consider friends and family a complementary therapy. Now, you won't read that in most books. It's probably not listed in any of the things that I've read about complementary therapies. But it's certainly equal to acupuncture or massage or anything else. Knowing you have people who can be there for you and who will go out of their way to learn to be there for you, and what that means, and what they shouldn't say to you and what they can say to you, and basically all they have to say to you is, 'How are you doing?' Don't get into platitudes like, 'God gives you as much as you can handle.' Or, 'Gee, you don't look sick.' People say some really bizarre things to you, and they mean well, but all of it has an impact on you. So you're learning all this in your first couple of months.

I think the biggest key to complementary therapies or integrative health is that it's something you can do to get back your life. You can't just rely on the doctors. You can't just rely on your caregivers. 'Patient', as Max Lerner writes in his book, *Wrestling with the Angel*, in Latin means 'to suffer.' And that was the old traditional definition. The relationship between doctors and patients was that you were the patient, you did what the doctor said, like you do what the mechanic says and the electrician says, and that's it. You can't operate like that.

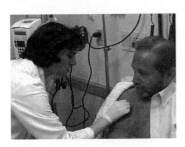 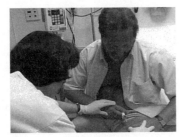 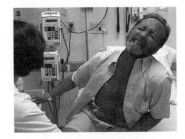

The problem was that I had not been given a menu of all the available choices that could help you get back your life. I had certain friends who said, you should try acupuncture or you should do this, and I wasn't closed-minded to it. I just didn't do it.

Then Joyce [Lenny's wife] and I went to see David Eisenberg [director of the Center for Alternative Medicine Research and Education at Beth Israel Deaconess Medical Center in Boston], and spent, I don't know, an hour with him, and he did a number of things. He gave me eight things to do that would help me prepare for the bone marrow transplant and then he gave me Michael Lerner's book, *Choices in Healing*, both of which were as key to my ability to prepare for this as anything. And what David—who is one of the pioneers in alternative complementary medicine in this country—told me to do, were very basic things. Exercise. Drink more water. Meditation. Acupuncture. Guided imagery. Massage therapy, and we're not talking about a backrub here. We're talking about serious therapeutic massage for people with chronic diseases. The only thing I didn't do was sleep more, because I really felt that if I was going to die, either before or after or during the transplant, I wasn't going to start giving away hours to go to sleep. I had a lot of things I wanted to do, and so I did seven out of the eight recommendations.

David tells me that he went home that night to his wife and said, 'I don't know if this guy got what I was telling him.' But I did get it. Most of my introduction and continuation of complementary therapies are people who David Eisenberg referred me to. And a couple others I picked up along the way. I began to work out with a trainer. That was one of the things David said.

I believe that Ken Anderson has saved my life and David Eisenberg has changed it. And it wasn't that David became my oncologist, or that he became my doctor. I didn't see him that often, but I did almost everything he said. What it did was open up to me the universe of complementary therapies, and through the acupuncturist he introduced me to, I learned more about herbs and vitamins, which I began to do at a major level.

My basic philosophy was what we in the Jewish community call the 'chicken soup' philosophy, which is that it can't hurt. So I talked to Ken Anderson and made sure he knew what I was doing, which, by the way, is fairly rare. According to the Eisenberg study, about 70 percent of people who do complementary therapies don't tell their doctors—they're afraid to tell their doctors—and I

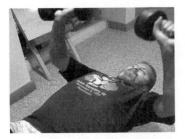 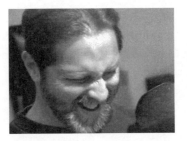 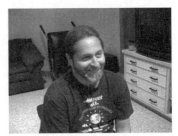

know of cases where doctors have accused them almost of traitorous behavior because they began to do complementary therapies.

What Eisenberg did was basically recommend to me standard complementary therapies which were very far out for some institutions, including Dana-Farber at the time, but they have anecdotal documentation, like 2,000 years worth of acupuncture. And, they don't hurt. The key is to make sure that they don't contradict the treatment you're on. There are some herbs, for instance, you can take that will contradict the good impact of the chemotherapy. It may serve to alleviate and assuage the bad impact, but if you're going through it, to take an herb that takes away the good impact doesn't make sense, because then you're just ravaging your body without it getting anything. So I started in the beginning with Ken, who didn't know very much about this but who was totally supportive, and we began to talk much more about these things: herbs and vitamins, basic vitamin C, echineacea which boosts your immunity system, milk thistle which helps purify your liver and kidney. There's a lot you can do to help deal with some of the bad side effects of chemotherapy and radiation, as well as just the ongoing problems of having cancer. All of this nutrition is a complementary therapy.

Nutrition, I knew nothing about, other than the food groups that I learned in third grade. No one told me that you could fight cancer with your fork. No one told me that there are certain foods you should eat when you're recovering or on chemotherapy or radiation that will help you, that will make you less sick, or less nauseous, or make you vomit less. They told me there were drugs, and in some cases, God bless drugs. You know there are times when all the faith and support in the world can't take the place of the drugs that we take. But there's a kind of inherent failure in a system that only prescribes you drugs to maintain your disease, because it's like, if the dam is bursting and all you keep doing is putting your finger in the dike, and it comes out other places, then you haven't fixed it. You're just fighting to preserve this weak status quo and that's what drugs do. You develop a dependency on some of these drugs, but one of the things about complementary therapies is that most of it is natural. Most of it is stuff you can do on your own. For some of it you need trained practitioners.

Nutrition. God, this is basic. When I was put on Prednisone [a steroid], it caused me great emotional stress, mood changes, pain in my bones when I was withdrawing from it. It caused me to have eating binges. If you have one cracker on Prednisone, you're going to eat the whole box. One chocolate chip cookie, and the bag's gone. Don't eat sugar. Don't eat salt. Have salad. There are a lot of things you can do nutritionally to help you deal with the effects of nausea and the hyperactivity you get from steroids and other things. And I didn't know that.

A support group—which I didn't understand and get into until after my transplant—is a critical part of recovery. It's at least a critical part of what I call complementary therapy, because in my support group, I began for the first time to realize that my insanity was legitimized. The things that you thought about, that no one who didn't have cancer could ever understand, these people have all been through. And the ability to talk to people who have been through what you have been through is a major boost. It doesn't alleviate your pain and it doesn't change your anxieties to a large degree, but it makes you feel that you're not crazy. Having a bone marrow stem cell transplant is not only as bad as you thought, it's worse. So hearing from people who had been through it made me stronger. It was also very important to go along with the other seven or eight things that I began to do. Mostly it gave me a little bit of a sense of empowerment that I could go and lift those weights.

Many people who are experiencing this aren't warned about fatigue by their doctors. I mean, they're warned that they'll be tired, but they're not given any tool to address it other than sleeping. Well, sleeping when you're really that tired is not always the best thing for you. You know, what's best for you might be to get going, get your system moving. That's what exercise does for you and I believe

"Nutrition, I knew nothing about, other than the food groups that I learned in third grade. No one told me that you could fight cancer with your fork."

Peter Churchill

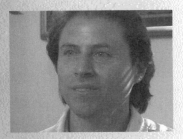

P
R
O
F
I
L
E

Therapeutic massage was one of the complementary therapies recommended to Lenny by Dr. David Eisenberg. Peter Churchill is a nationally certified massage and bodywork therapist, who also teaches at Harvard Medical School. He has worked with Lenny for the past three years.

"Lenny has come almost every week for the whole time he's had the cancer, so we've developed quite a connection. What I first do with people is to establish a healing partnership where we're a team together. When we come together, we create a sacred space. Sometimes we talk, sometimes we listen to music, sometimes we're just quiet, but we're entering into what I call the 'healing equation,' where his openness, and my skill and openness meet together, and then some magic happens.

"In Lenny's case, we've gone through times of him being in absolute pain where he can barely walk through the door; other days where he's feeling fantastic and it seems like everything has been cleared out of his body and he's free of the cancer; and times when he's had radiation or chemotherapy and is in agony afterwards, or in despair when he's found out bad news about a particular moment in the whole process.

"When I was young, I spent a lot of time in nature, and I began to learn to be still and listen. And then as I began to work with people, I noticed I could listen and be quiet and feel them in a profound way. I could feel their heart; I could feel if it was hurt. I could feel if a part of their body was injured; I could feel if somewhere inside, one of their organ systems was not working right. And so that same listening, that same stillness that I found in nature, I was then able to translate into working with people.

"In my own life, I practice all that I recommend to other people. I find a way every day to stay open to spirit so I can listen and feel effectively. Then when I touch somebody or work with them, that balance

"What I first do with people is to establish a healing partnership where we're a team together...when we come together, it's a sacred space."

of life-force comes into them and can help them. I don't say much about this when I work with people. Sometimes they ask me what's happening because they feel a warmth and tingling, or they notice they're getting better all of a sudden.

"So this, of course, would make most scientists and doctors immediately skeptical, but I want to talk like this because it is real. This process is genuine. It helps people, and it's not quackery. There are laws to how this hands-on healing process works, but they're different. They're more subtle. Most of the machines that have been made to detect energy are still too crude to detect the more subtle life-energy I'm talking about. It's just as invisible as electricity, but it's tangible and people feel it.

"You have to open your heart to have it really do much good for you. I've had people come in who say, 'I heard you did this remarkable healing work with somebody, do it to me,' as if it's an order, and it often doesn't work because their own heart hasn't opened. I've particularly seen this if people are referred here and they come against their will, if they don't really want to do it but they feel obliged to, or are merely curious. Often, unless that person goes through a process where they ask for help and open their own heart, nothing profound occurs. It's as if we are only meeting at the physical level. Real healing always has to happen in the heart and in the energy system of a person—and that includes their body—but it has to happen in these dimensions to be effective.

"Even with an oncologist who's giving chemotherapy, he's giving a physical substance, but the way it heals is that it does something to the cellular energy of the person. It kills cancer cells so that the per-

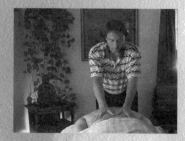
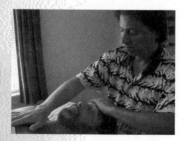
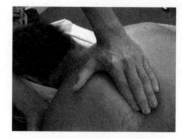

son's life-force and vitality can get strong again, and then it is the life-force that heals them. No drug in the world ever heals anybody, and no healer who puts his hands on someone ever heals anybody. Both are just using different ways to open the energy and life-force in a person, and then assisting that life-force to heal them.

"One way or another, everybody needs to go deep in their life. They need to go deeper, beyond the superficial daily ordinariness of life, and illnesses often are a catalyst to go deep. Many times people will say after they've gone through the cancer that it was a gift. Not in the midst of their pain, not that it's good that it hurts and that their life is suffering, but something occurs where their heart opens again and they begin to appreciate what's really important. And they face death, and when you face death, you become a deeper person.

"Healing can happen very quickly. Sometimes it's a life-long ordeal. It can be very quick, though, when you go to that deep place. And other times you can go to that place and the process goes on and on, and it just breaks your heart, like with Lenny. We go to that place again and again. He's fighting for his life every day. The miracle hasn't happened where the cancer has just lifted away. We have to stay in it and go through it day after day, and we don't know what will happen. We just try to do our best with this healing work.

"Lenny's never given up. His spirit stays strong, and if it gets a little low, I try to boost him up so that we don't lose hope. Any time I've ever worked with somebody who loses their spirit and gives up, the end is usually near and they slip away. It's incredible how important that is, and I know anybody who practices medicine knows that. But I think a physician can get caught up in the tests and the drugs and the surgeries and forget how delicate the balance of hope can be, and how important the spirit is, and how much it can mean to just reach out and hold somebody's hand and touch them with love."

"No drug in the world ever heals anybody, and no healer who puts his hands on someone ever heals anybody. Both are just using different ways to open the energy and life-force in a person, and then assisting that life-force to heal them."

that firmly, no matter what status of cancer you have, unless you're in your final days, or if you're elderly. But there have been tests that show that elderly people on walkers or crutches or who are bedridden who begin to lift weights, five-pound weights, within a few weeks will get rid of, in many cases, those crutches and those walkers, because you're getting your system going again.

The tendency of people when they're sick is to go to bed. The tendency of people who are in pain is to lay there, take painkillers, drugs, and wait for it to go away, and the tendency of many doctors is to give you all those pills and tell you to go to bed. What you learn through complementary therapies is, that's not the best thing to do. I learned that in dealing with this terrible disease and the feelings of depression and exhaustion and pain that you have, that exercise and meditation and acupuncture make a significant difference. It doesn't make the cancer go away. It doesn't cure you from the cancer, but it helps you deal with the other stuff you're going through. I mean, you are waging war on your body and you've got to have a strong spiritual base, whether you're an atheist or whether you're religious—Catholic, Protestant, Jew or Muslim, you've got to have some base of belief system, value system, beliefs that will get you through this stuff.

You also have to have a strong emotional base, which is family and friends. Joyce and my parents spent every day with me in the hospital when I was in isolation; they were allowed in with their coats and gowns and masks and stuff. My kids were not allowed in, which was the worst part of that isolation period, but I had a couple of friends that came every single night. Every night, no matter what was going on in their lives. Three-quarters of the nights I was unconscious, and I might wake up for a minute and I'd look around, and they'd be watching *Seinfeld*, or they'd be talking, but they were there. That was a big boost, because being alone really maximizes your fear.

I want to know that Dana-Farber offers acupuncture, massage and other things in addition to chemotherapy and radiation. But, more important, I want to know that my oncologist is not only going to tell me that I'm about to have chemotherapy, radiation, steroid treatment, and go through this horrible thing; but they're also going to say, by the way, in our community, there are respected acupuncturists, massage therapists, guided therapy people, people who can help you deal with all the aspects of cancer that affect you as a full person.

I learned it the hard way, but I think most of us learn it the hard way. And the one thing that a cancer diagnosis does is reduce you to your lowest common denominator. I don't care if you're the president of the United States, or the head of a big company, or a teacher, or a public works person. When you're diagnosed with cancer, you are stripped of titles, you're stripped of previous power, ideas of power, illusions of control. And if we're not told in that early stage that there are things you can do for yourself, you are less able to cope with this thing because cancer is a disease that doesn't just affect your body, it affects your mind, it affects your soul, it affects your heart. It affects every relationship you have. It affects your entire community. You know, you are the CEO or the president of your life. Well, you get diagnosed with one of these diseases and you're the stockboy. You forget being the CEO of your life. And you're dependent on everybody, and if you're an independent person, to learn to be dependent is a very, very, very hard thing.

I think what bothered me most through this process is the kind of 'wait for it to get worse' mentality that most hospitals promote. You can't expect your hospitals to become your psycho-social support system totally. I mean, your hospital, your doctor, your nurse and your administrators and the wonderful people so committed to helping you get better, are not coming into your living room when you have to sit down and tell your kids. For me, the worst part of this whole experience is telling the kids and then seeing the impact that this has on your kids. I don't care how old you are. Seeing the impact it has on my parents has not been very pleasurable either. But telling the kids was the hardest thing that I've ever done in my life.

Living with cancer is hard for them, because for me one of the worst things is that I don't want to be thought of—I don't want to be remembered anyway—as a person who was sick. I don't want my kids to think of me as being

POWER

"When you're diagnosed with cancer, you're stripped of titles, you're stripped of previous power, ideas of power, illusions of control. And if we're not told in that early stage that there are things you can do for yourself, you are less able to cope with this thing."

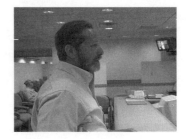

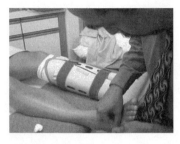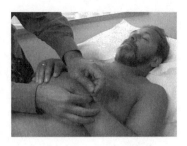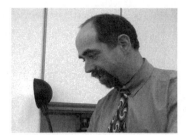

sick. When you lose your hair and you're lying in bed and you're sleeping half the day, I don't care if you get up out of the bed and do the treadmill—you're still in bed most of the time. Or when you're in isolation and you can't see them, and that's really unraveling for them and for you. And there are things you can learn on how to do that. One of the things I think that was important for my kids was to see me get up out of bed, early on, and get on the treadmill. I may have looked horrible. I may have looked half-dead. They knew I was weak. They knew what we had told them, and they intuitively know more because kids are like cats and dogs. They can sense nervousness even if you put on bravado.

For me, the most incredible example of the benefits of acupuncture besides the fatigue and the pain reduction is this: I had acute conjunctivitis, just a few months ago. I literally had burning, itchy, red, caked eyes. I'd wake up in the night, couldn't open my eyes, they were like glued together. I put on the antibiotic salve that my doctor told me to do, and after two days that hadn't done anything. I went to acupuncture and he did three needles here and three needles here and it was gone within an hour: the itching, the burning, and the red. Is that a clinical trial? I can't tell you that it is. But it works. For me, and for a lot of other people.

At all levels, I think the complementary therapy piece is your first real grab back at self-determination and empowerment and whatever word you call it. It gives you at least some sense that you can do stuff for yourself. You're not totally helpless. It doesn't change the emphasis or the reliance on your doctors and on the care, but it does improve and enhance your reliance on yourself. So you have the medical side, and you have the physical side—the ups and downs, the exercise as well as the side effects. The other part is spiritual. The other complementary therapy. There was a headline in *The Boston Globe* that said prayer is good for patients, or something like that. To me that was as stupid a head-line as it could possibly get because it so stated the obvious. It's like water helps a thirsty person. Food helps a hungry person. Of course it does.

I should be able to walk into any cancer institution in this country and find not only the directory to chemotherapy, radiation, steroid treatments and various other and sundry drugs, but I want them to also be saying to patients like me, 'Okay, we asked you how you're doing under the chemo. Have you seen the acupuncturist yet?' Do you know that acupuncture has been found by the NCI [National Cancer Institute] or the NIH [National Institutes of Health] to actually be proven to reduce fatigue and nausea after chemotherapy? Do you know that eating certain vegetables helps restore key nutrients to your body, antioxidants, etc., which are cancer retardant?'

Some of the doctors who are most committed and most sincere are afraid of complementary therapies, because they can't prove that it works. I respect that reason, but I don't accept it as a reason not to share with people. Can you tell me anybody that you've ever known that doesn't feel better after a massage? There's no harm that can be done unless you have bones that are in very frag-ile condition like I do, and then you have to tell the massage person to work on muscles and not go near bones. There are ways around this.

The bottom line for me is that, in all of this journey that I've been on which is so full of fears and legitimate fears—it's one of those times that when you're paranoid, somebody really is out to get you, this isn't something that's in your mind—you can't distinguish anymore between an ache that's natural and an ache related to your cancer. Once you've been thrown off that illusion of con-trol and that illusion of health, everything's related, and there will be some who don't understand this.

There will be some who live with us patients, work with us patients, who say, 'There he goes again. He just stumbled. He must think it's cancer. What's the matter with that guy.' Hey, that's our struggle. But there are reasons for it. We've been put into one of the worst situations possible. I know that when I was about to go into isolation, I talked to two friends of mine who are holocaust survivors, and I thought of them and Nathan Sharansky and Nelson Mandela in their little cells for years on end, and I said, 'How did you do this? How did you survive this?' And holocaust survivor Elie Wiesel told me, 'One day at a time. Don't think too much about the past. Don't think about tomorrow. One day at a time.' And that's an important piece, too.

To be told you have an incurable cancer—which is what I was told, which apparently still remains the case—that's a lot to take, and you've got to pull at whatever strings you have and some of it's prayer and faith. Faith in people. Faith in God. Some of it's very practical things like exercise and meditation and acupuncture. Certainly some of it's in the chemotherapy and radiation and ongoing treatment from your oncologist.

I really believe that it's a failure of Western medicine not to integrate all of this into it. We patients are doing it on our own, and we're lost out there. We need a coach. And maybe the coach can't be the doctor who has the primary responsibility for your dealing with your illness, but your caregiver has to be in a partnership with you. Your caregiver, your doctor, your nurse, has to be open to this. And, it's not one versus the other. Anybody who just does complementary therapies and doesn't do conventional therapies, that's their decision, that's their right, it's their life. I would empathize with anyone who was looking at a reduced life span and makes a decision not to do conventional treatments, because of all the pain and reducing of quality of life. I would be the last person to judge that person, but if you want to continue living and have a quality of life, and feel like I do—that I owe it to my kids, my family, to do everything I possibly can—then here's this tremendous resource.

Doctors should be introducing us to that resource. Nurses should be introducing us to that resource. I mean, I know of cases where doctors and nurses who know about it, hide it, because they're afraid they're not going to be treated seriously by their colleagues. We have to work on this together. I've relapsed twice now. And I've been through the transplant. I've done all these complementary therapies. I still have cancer. It's a drag. I'm bored with it. I need other challenges in my life. But I'm very fortunate that I'm still around.

FAITH

"To be told you have an incurable cancer—which is what I was told, which apparently still remains the case—that's a lot to take and you've got to pull at whatever strings you have, and some of it's prayer and faith."

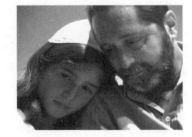

I know people who died during their transplant. I'm lucky to be around. I'm lucky to have the kind of care I get at the Dana-Farber, but I don't think that anything on its own is what's kept me going. I think a lot of it is what different people have done for me and what I've done for myself, and the best thing I've done for myself, besides refuse to quit—which is not easy to do sometimes—is to do the complementary therapies, because in almost every case it makes me feel better physically, emotionally. It makes me stronger, and if you're planning to run this marathon, then you've got to do everything you can.

You've got all that stuff going on. I think you've got to do something positive, assertive for yourself, and that's getting on the treadmill and that's lifting the weights. And every time I lifted those weights, I felt like I was striking a blow against cancer. Guided imagery, which is something you're taught, too, that's proven to reduce pain. Those guys who walk over the hot coals in their bare feet, that's a form of guided imagery. I don't know all that much about how they do it, but they do it, and they don't burn their feet. How's that done? What capacities do we have within ourselves, emotionally, spiritually, mentally, physically, that can get by all this?

People can come up with any images they want. It could be oceans, it could be flowers, I don't care, whatever works, but guided imagery is important. When you're feeling most vulnerable, when you're feeling most afraid, when you are lying there writhing in pain, when you are vomiting over yourself and you can't control your body parts—I won't go into all the gory details of all these things that all of us cancer patients go through. I guess my bottom line on all of it is, you live with it and you try to do the best with it when you have these relapses or you have continued problems, or for those lucky enough to go into remission, it may come back.

T
H
E
R
A
P
I
E
S

"The best thing I've done for myself, besides refuse to quit— which is not easy to do sometimes—is to do the complementary therapies, because in almost every case it makes me feel better."

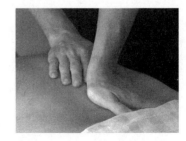

I've questioned this. I've been told by my doctor that everything came back to a level it was before my transplant, and I sat there for a day or so, and I said, does all this matter? I mean, does it really matter? I've done acupuncture every week. I've gone to massage therapy every week where he massages my thymus gland which kicks off more T-cells and reduces my pain, and I've done it. I've done it all. I work out. All this stuff. How come I'm still sick? How come I still have cancer? How come it's not cured?

I sift through that process. But I didn't stop doing any of those things. Because I'm not going to try getting through this unless I'm doing everything I can. And, secondly, it does help. Who knows how much worse I haven't gotten because I'm doing this stuff. It doesn't cure cancer. But, I'll tell you something, three years of repeated chemotherapy hasn't cured the cancer, either. Neither has the radiation I've gone through. Neither has this horrible transplant I went through. None of it cured it.

So, for those who are cynics, doubters, particularly doctors who say, 'Well, it's not going to cure it': Hey, guys, you're running an institution that's keeping us, hopefully, alive for a long time, but how are you doing it? Chemotherapy, radiation, and how come we still have cancer?

My doctor told me everything in the world there was to know about multiple myeloma, and thank God, he was open to me bringing all the other stuff in. But I really do want the day to come where I'm going to walk in there and they're going to give me that book that says, 'Okay, here's the resources of this hospital and it includes yoga, meditation, etc.,' because that's what they owe us. We're paying good money.

And, the other thing they owe us, by the way, is to get insurance companies to begin to pay reimbursements for this, because even if you're insured, the out-of-pocket expenses you incur in vitamins and herbs, the basic vitamins, they're expensive. There's got to be a system in which doctors will work with you to move the insurance companies, which Ken Anderson did. He wrote some of the strongest letters you could possibly write, and said to my insurance company that he felt that massage therapy, acupuncture, and exercise were as important to my ability to cope with cancer as the chemotherapy and radiation was. Now, you don't get any better than that. It still took a year and a half to get reimbursed, but I did, and I think that insurance companies have to begin to move in that direction. Otherwise, if you don't have great insurance, or don't have a great doctor, you're stuck.

5 LENNY'S STORY PART 2
CANCER AND THE SEARCH FOR HEALING

During our interviews with them, several of Lenny's healthcare providers referred to the fact that he has had access to the very best, both in his conventional medical treatment and complementary therapies. Lenny knows that, too, which is why he has made it his new life mission to bring awareness of these therapies to as many people as possible. In his view, even very conservative, traditional treatment centers—cancer institutes, hospitals, and health clinics—should make information and advice about more unconventional therapies readily available to their patients.

In the next chapter, we hear directly from Dr. David Eisenberg about the measured approach he recommends to cancer patients—indeed, to anyone interested in exploring complementary therapies. Lenny's oncologist, Dr. Ken Anderson, demonstrates the open and curious mind that he brought to his treatment plan for Lenny, and Michael Lerner, co-founder of the Commonweal Cancer Help Program, explores the important difference between "curing" and "healing."

DAVID EISENBERG

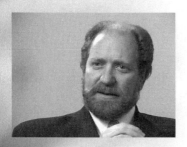

Eight months into his battle against multiple myeloma, Lenny Zakim decided to begin exploring complementary therapies. A mutual friend steered him to David Eisenberg, M.D., a conventionally trained doctor who spent two years during medical school as an exchange student in the Far East, where he explored treatments used in traditional Chinese medicine. As director of the Center for Alternative Medicine Research and Education at Beth Israel Deaconess Medical Center in Boston, Dr. Eisenberg no longer sees private patients; his current mission is to discover which complementary therapies are truly useful. Lenny often says that his oncologist, Ken Anderson, saved his life, but that David Eisenberg changed it. It is a tribute that Dr. Eisenberg is reluctant to accept.

EISENBERG: Lenny changed Lenny's life. I did my best to give him some advice, to try to challenge him to make use of all the conventional, allopathic, biomedical, technological expertise he had access to, and also to look at the other less conventional things that might be useful for Lenny.

I have to emphasize that there's no prescription which can be generalized from Lenny Zakim to every person with cancer, but I did challenge Lenny because he asked me for advice. He told me he was going to prepare for a bone marrow transplant. He described how he was working a million hours a week, how he was out of shape, how he was not eating a balanced, let alone an ideal, diet. He had a lot of, in my mind, curious if not erroneous ideas about taking handfuls of vitamins and supplements and herbs, which might or might not put him at risk. He was dropped into a jungle without a map, and he was looking for somebody with a map and a flashlight. So I was the fortunate one to meet him in the jungle. If I put on my conventional, primary care doctor hat, I did for

Lenny what I would do for anybody, even if I didn't have an interest in alternative or complementary non-allopathic medicine. I would say, 'Let's start with the basics. What do you eat? Do you exercise? Have you ever exercised? Do you know the first thing about a balanced diet? Or a routine graduated exercise program? What do you expect from the alternative therapies?'

A lot of people have unrealistic expectations. They see them as magic bullets that will cure them. I needed to see if Lenny thought these were the cure, or parts of his journey to maximize whatever health and potential he had left. He was depressed. He was anxious. He was frightened. Was he getting any kind of help, professional or lay help, to just process the emotional roller-coaster ride of facing a terminal disease? I think any good primary care physician or subspecialist wants to check in with the patient and see if they're getting some help. Nobody can process that alone or exclusively, I think, with the biased opinions of loved ones who have very conflicted interests. So: diet, exercise. What medicines was he taking? What herbs and vitamins was he contemplating taking? Which ones, if any, have any scientific basis, and which ones were sort of shots in the dark based on anecdote and hyperbole and fantasy and hope? My job, simply, was to say to Lenny, 'Time out. Where are you on the conventional side? What alternative things are you even remotely interested in or already dabbling in? And how do you put this together?' Not everyone likes massage. Some people don't like being touched. Some people would never dream of having acupuncture needles put into their bodies. They're phobic of needles. For others, they're waiting for the chance for a physician to say, 'I'd like you to try that, because I think it's powerful,' and it may well be.

Let me emphasize there's no magic formula, so let's start with basics. People need, I think, to figure out what's going on conventionally. What is their diagnosis? What is the conventional recommendation? And have they maximized that? Lenny was blessed with access to one of the finest medical institutions on the planet, and in Ken Anderson, one of the greatest physicians and most knowledgeable human beings on his particular illness. He got that right. And his job was to maximize every drop of that. My hat is off to Ken Anderson and his colleagues who have delivered the state of the science, high-tech, bio-tech, chemotherapeutic, radiation, bone marrow approach to a horrible disease.

J U N G L E

"[Lenny] was dropped into a jungle without a map, and he was looking for somebody with a map and a flashlight."

Lenny also wanted to look at other options, and I think that's the next step. At what point are the conventional options either exhausted or unacceptable? So he was coming to me to look at the other, less conventional, often unstudied options. My job was to explore with him his thoughts, which ones were really off-base and how he could integrate one or more of the alternative complementary therapies with conventional care. But not as an either/or, as *both*. Now, he was in a unique situation, anticipating a bone marrow transplant. He was not like a woman about to receive chemotherapy for breast cancer saying, 'Which herb or vitamin do I take now?' Or not like the patient who had already failed to respond to a very aggressive course of therapy and was in pain, saying, 'What can I take for my pain?' These are all different situations. This is what I mean by the improvisational dance.

Lenny was one of the fortunate few anticipating a big gamble. He had to prepare for a bone marrow transplant. So when I met him and his wife I said, 'You've got a marathon. You've got to maximize everything you've got. You have to become a star athlete. You have to gain focus and control of your mind and your body. You are going to go through hell and back. Are you ready?' And it was obvious he was working too hard. He was not processing a lot of the emotional issues. He was not getting prepared. He was not eating well. He thought he would just sort of stop, have the bone marrow transplant and that was it.

So my focus with Lenny was getting prepared. And in that conversation after diet and exercise and mental health issues—which are routine, these are not alternative—we talked about vitamins and supplements. We talked about which ones are known to have any relevance to his particular problem and which ones may be dangerous. I think the role of a clinician in these circumstances is not to be a blatant advocate or skeptic, but to give the best advice they can for the individual patient as to what's a judicious integration. What makes sense out of this enormous black bag for any patient, from the conventional or the alternative realm?

M A R A T H O N

"When I met Lenny and his wife, I said, 'You've got a marathon. You've got to maximize everything you've got. You have to become a star athlete. You have to gain focus and control of your mind and your body. You are going to go through hell and back. Are you ready?'"

A lot of my job was telling Lenny, 'Don't do that. Or don't do that with 19 other things and expect to make sense of what just happened when you feel better or worse.' A lot of people who pursue alternative therapies when dropped in that dark jungle without a map, do it all at once. And then they feel better or worse, and they don't know whether the herbs or the acupuncture or the massage or the meditation exhausted them more or made them feel better. There's no sense of causality. They can't make an association, because they just haven't used common sense to add them one at a time. So with Lenny, I said, 'Let's focus on a symptom. Whether it's fatigue or pain, let's just focus on one symptom and that will be your map.' Anybody with cancer can do that, particularly somebody who has a symptom. If people keep a little diary every day about their pain or their fatigue or their nausea or their lack of focus or their fear, that's the baseline. That's the map. They can show it to their doctor, their spouse, or their child, or their mother. And then methodically they can think about adding one behavioral change or intervention at a time, because if you add three at a time and you feel better, you don't know which one or ones helped. More importantly, if you add three at a time, and any one of them involves an herb or a vitamin or a supplement, and you feel nauseated or have a rash or have some unexplainable physiologic change, we don't know. Was it the herb, the vitamin, its interaction with your chemotherapy? In other words, if there are too many changing parts at once, you can't make logical sense as to what caused you to feel better or worse. Keep it simple: one thing at a time, focusing on one or two very reliable indicators of how one is feeling.

Lenny kept a diary. Lenny added one or at most two things at once. He was very hard to chain down. He's a race horse, Lenny. But little by little he added each of these components and he, unlike most people, loved them all. That's Lenny's personality. They were all beneficial for Lenny. Meditation, exercise, a trainer, balanced diet, much less fat. Some vitamins but not excessive vitamins. Acupuncture. Not everybody would seek all of those; not everybody would add all of those. That's okay. The other thing he did, very wisely, was to discuss it openly with his oncologist. I made him promise not to set this up as an either/or proposition. This is trying to create an integrated approach that maximizes his chances. So he did these things to prepare for his bone marrow transplant with the full knowledge of his clinicians, who, to their credit, said, 'Fine. We applaud you for losing the weight, getting in shape, trying the acupuncture, doing stress reduction with massage. Fine.' It didn't conflict with what they had to say.

Now let's take a bizarre hypothetical example. If Lenny had seen an acupuncturist who wanted to prescribe herbs while he was getting chemotherapy or radiation, there would be a conflict. I think that conflict should be openly discussed. I feel very strongly that 'don't ask and don't tell' does not work when it comes to complementary therapies, particularly for people with serious illness on prescription drugs. There has to be an open triangular conversation between the patient, their conventional provider, and their complementary or alternative provider. Otherwise, the patient is trapped without an ally or a guide. They don't know whose side to take. So when there is conflict, it's best for the doctor to sit and discuss it, and ultimately bow to the patient. But the physician's job, I think, is to say, 'This is how I see it. I want you to know it.'

I've never met a patient in years of taking these shared journeys who didn't appreciate the discussion of the conflict. I think they want that. In fact, I think the country is crying out for conventionally trained doctors and nurses and physical therapists from all backgrounds and specialties who are knowledgeable about both. Not necessarily expert in both, but sufficiently knowledgeable about both and sufficiently nonjudgmental to imagine that there's an integrated approach that may be beneficial for some people some of the time.

The definition of complementary or alternative medicine, which I'm partially to blame for, is from the *New England Journal of Medicine* article that I wrote with colleagues in 1993, that looked at these things as therapies that are not commonly taught in U.S. medical schools or commonly available in U.S. hospitals. Acupuncture, chiropractic, massage, homeopathy, herbs. It's a lousy definition. The field is growing bigger.

About a year ago, a patient on a panel said to me, 'Dr. Eisenberg, respectfully, I disagree with your definition.' She was almost exactly my age. She had lived with chronic lymphoma for 20 years. She said, 'I'm alive because of chemotherapy and surgery and radiation. I owe my life to the science of biomedicine. But I've also used all of the complementary and alternative therapies you discussed. I've used acupuncture and meditation and massage and herbs, and even energy healing and prayer. I have used them all. My definition of alternative therapies, Dr. Eisenberg, is that these are the therapies which for 20 years I've had to pay for out-of-pocket and could never feel comfortable discussing with my oncologist. That's the definition.' I think it's unacceptable that people with cancer or any chronic illness feel that they can't discuss it with their doctors. We have the responsibility to fix that, to become better educated about these things, so we can have the conversation and welcome it and make them feel that no matter how much we may disagree or find it unsubstantiated by scientific research, controlled trials, hard evidence, we owe it to them to make a place to have the conversation.

And as Lenny has made it clear to the institution that cares for him and the larger community, it is unacceptable that patients with cancer don't have a place to go to say, 'What else should I take? And what else should I avoid? What will interact with my standard therapy?' And the unspoken question: 'Will you, my conventional caregivers, think less of me for asking you this question? Have I ruined our relationship now, by asking you what you think about macrobiotics or meditation or laying on of hands?' I think patients shouldn't be put in that position. We should make a space for them to ask. Having said all of this, I need you to know that I'm not sure which, if any, of these things has or will help Lenny Zakim. In the absence of controlled scientific experiments, we don't know which is useful and which is useless; which is being pushed by a market with an insatiable desire to fix, to cure, to relieve, to live forever. A large generation of people, particularly my age, want it all, and won't accept failure, and won't accept disease or incapacitation or death. We need to figure out which are real and which are hyperbole and hype and charlatanism.

That's the work I do and that colleagues around the country are doing. We have a center, the Center for Alternative Medicine Research and Education, here at Beth Israel Deaconess Medical Center and Harvard Medical School. We're devoted to distinguishing use*ful* from use*less*; for clarifying which work, which improve outcomes and which do not; which decrease costs, which increase costs. Then how do you measure those costs, and quality of life and satisfaction or bottom line. But those are research questions, and I'd hate to be viewed by Lenny or anyone else as a blind advocate. I'm not. I just want to know what's good for people like Lenny Zakim, because I feel morally it's unacceptable to

R E L I E V E

"In the absence of controlled scientific experiments, we don't know which [complementary therapy] is useful and which is useless; which is being pushed by a market with an insatiable desire to fix, to cure, to relieve, to live forever. We need to figure out which are real and which are hyperbole and hype and charlatanism."

have no script to give them. I'd love in every institution in this country for there to be at least one physician in every key department, whether it's oncology or orthopedics or cardiology, one M.D., one nurse specialist, who's comfortable in both domains, who's bilingual, who can say, 'Come, let's talk. Let's talk about both. Neither of them scares me. I can refer you either way. Let's talk.'

We need that. That's part of the future of American health care, because the market is demanding it. People deserve and demand responsible advice. They don't want to do this secretly. I don't think anybody in their right mind wants to do something that puts them at risk for an interaction between their drug and their herb or vitamin. I don't think anybody wants to do anything that know-ingly, knowledgeably, interacts with their physician's recommendations. They want people who can guide them on both levels of the terrain. It's rocky out there with chronic disease, so they need people who can speak both languages.

The other thing is, Lenny is unique because of his position in society. This is not meant as a criticism. Lenny knows a lot of people. Lenny has access to the best. We can't afford to have complementary and alternative medicine made accessible only to people with the connections of a Lenny Zakim or the finances of a rich individual. That's unacceptable. The alternative therapies that work cannot only be for rich, white people, and the research can't only involve upper-class white people. As these therapies become more and more attractive to the business community and are made available as products, it's unacceptable for them to be made available to people with more disposable income, to not involve individuals from minorities, inner-city populations, people on Medic-aid or Medicare. If these things are beneficial, they must be made accessible to those individuals as well. Otherwise, it's just another vehicle to create a two-class system of health care. And we've done that too many times.

Lenny wants this to be made available to everybody with cancer. He is on a mis-sion from God to see this through. He's changed a lot of minds in this insti-tution by saying to them, 'You cannot have the next 10,000 people with cancer proceed without advice from people in white coats and stethoscopes as to their diet. Whether group therapy or individual psychotherapy or meditation is help-ful. Which vitamins or herbs. When they need an acupuncturist, who to see.

MISSION

"Lenny wants this to be made available to everybody with cancer. He is on a mission from God to see this through."

Whether massage is helpful.' He will not allow conventional institutions to duck those questions.

Our hospital, the Beth Israel Deaconess Medical Center, is committed to developing that information for such patients, is committed to developing integrated models of care. Not marginalized. Not a little clinic in the corner, far away. In the belly of the hospital, bringing people from each of the disciplines: oncology, cardiology, orthopedics, neurology, where the chronically ill are, putting them together with chiropractors, acupuncturists, massage therapists, exercise trainers, mind/body experts. We need to demarginalize this and demystify it and figure out, how do you build an integrated unit for people with cancer or chronic musculoskeletal pain, and give them advice, and give them services, and refer them to licensed practitioners. We're going to do that. I hope all the hospitals in the country do it, too. Because I think that's what people want. It in no way takes anything away from the gifts of science and medicine and surgery and antibiotics. They are not either/or. They have to be integrated. That's Lenny's message, I think. And he's going to try to make it happen as fast as possible.

BODY & SOUL: I have a question about the desperation that people feel when they're faced with a cancer diagnosis. Many people have said to me, 'It's the worst thing I've ever heard in my life.' People are suddenly changed, transformed by those words, and they're vulnerable as a result.

EISENBERG: I can't imagine anything that would make one feel more desperate and vulnerable than being told there's a high possibility you're going to die from this disease. I think the fears that go through people's minds are not so much the pain but the uncertainty. Abandonment, the burden they place on others, and the lack of control, lack of involvement, lack of participation. But, you know, I think in that vulnerability we often find people who seek magical

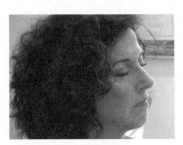 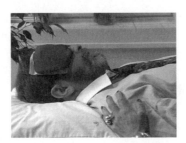 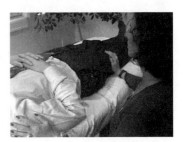

cures, or who pay a lot of money to individuals who say, 'I'm the only one who can deliver this to you.' If it sounds too good to be true, it probably is. There are charlatans, and there are unethical people, and there are quacks. There are also well-intentioned individuals who believe that they have the power to cure cancer, but this is not the way to solve the problem.

Part of my work and the work of others committed to the rigorous scientific evaluation of these therapies is to do all of this in the sunlight, under careful evaluation, open to every possibility. What if? What if there is a magical cure? We should at least understand it and evaluate it. That's sort of why the NIH originally set up the Office of Alternative Medicine—now, the National Center for Complementary and Alternative Medicine—to explore the anomalous, unexpected event. Having said that, I think the common element between what the NIH set in motion and what people like me and my most skeptical colleagues share is the understanding that science is the ally here. It's not the bogey man. To evaluate these things fairly and rigorously with everybody at the table—practitioner, skeptic, basic scientist, advocate, policymaker, insurance carrier, businessman, manufacturer—that's the way we do good science. And we need more resources to throw at this science.

My favorite Chinese proverb—I spent almost two years in China—is, literally, 'Real gold does not fear the heat of even the hottest fire.' We have all the tools at our disposal to distinguish useful from useless anti-cancer treatments. We should do that. We should test them in large numbers under the scrutiny of skeptical scientists in our most conservative medical institutions. It may sound counter-intuitive, but from where I sit, the people who are advocates for complementary medicine and the professions of chiropractic, acupuncture, herbal medicine, manufacturers of supplements, many of them want to shake hands and say, 'Let's do this together. We are not afraid. We believe in what we do. Test us. Just test us.' So I think as we come to the end of a century and enter a new millennium, for the very first time we have the tools of science to distinguish useful from useless, and the political will to bring the advocates and the skeptics to one table and say, 'We're going to figure this out. And we're going to create the script for the next people with cancer or chronic problems. We're going to educate clinicians to have a responsible but evidence-based conversation. That's what the public wants. Not just in this country, but globally. All of these issues are global issues. So we'll do it.'

What if some of this works *because* people believe in it? My own interest in this field grows out of a consciousness in 1973, when I was 17 years old, that said China is opening up. I read this dusty book, *The Yellow Emperor's Canon of Internal Medicine*, 24 centuries old, and it impressed me on two levels. It said prevention is always superior to intervention. To administer to a disease that has already occurred is like one who would dig a well after growing thirsty or one who would build weapons after engaging in battle. Wouldn't these things be too late? And secondly, it said the way one lives one's life: physically, diet, exercise, sexual activity, but also psychically, emotionally, spiritually, all have an impact on health, illness, and the progression of disease. So I was attracted to this question of whether the mind impacts the body, but now I don't know the degree to which it's important and for whom. That's why I went into research and became a card-carrying member of the skeptical medical community first. In which instances is it the herb, the needle, the pill? And in which instances is it the *belief* in the herb, the needle, the pill? When it's the latter, when it's the belief or the expectation that the therapy will help me, how does that happen? How is it possible that for some people—maybe Lenny, maybe not—it is the belief, the passion that says this is going to help me which becomes the physiologic self-fulfilling prophecy that I am helped. What if it is placebo? Placebo is 'to please.' What if the notion that will please me and help me is enough for some people, that they are wired in such a way that it changes their immune system or their nervous system or their endocrine system?

Twenty years from now, long after I'm done with my work, the basic scientists behind me, I hope, will begin to make sense of how belief, expectation, and emotion could have an impact physiologically to make a dent in serious illness. That's hard science. Which genes are turned on and off by a belief and expectation, or by a dietary supplement? That's where all the work my colleagues and I are doing is handed off to the scientists behind us, to understand why. That could be a real contribution to biology and the future of medicine. It's not either/or. It starts with the premise that in some people belief, expectation, patient-provided magic or fear can increase or decrease the effect of the therapy. I believe that. If I could understand it, I'd have made something of my life.

KEN ANDERSON

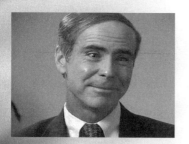

Ken Anderson, M.D., is the oncologist Lenny Zakim credits with saving his life so far, following his diagnosis of multiple myeloma in January of 1995. An estimated 15,000 Americans are diagnosed every year with this rare form of bone marrow cancer, which normally affects people 60 years of age and older. With chemotherapy and sometimes radiation therapy, most patients may do well for three to four years, according to Dr. Anderson. So far, however, there is no known cure. Until he met Lenny Zakim, Dr. Anderson says he knew almost nothing about complementary therapies for cancer patients.

BODY & SOUL: How do complementary or alternative therapies work with your traditional therapies?

ANDERSON: I think complementary therapies play a very important role in the treatment of patients with cancer and other illnesses as well. They're not in any way a substitute for therapies that we utilize to treat the underlying diseases, whatever they may be. In this instance, with multiple myeloma, in Lenny's case, we've used traditional chemotherapy and we've even used very high doses of chemotherapy and stem cell transplantation. So we've used not only conventional, traditional medicine approaches, but we've used research approaches within traditional medicine as well. Where complementary therapies come in, in my opinion, is that they are very much a part of the whole treatment plan. They make it much more readily achievable to carry out our traditional chemotherapy treatments. In this instance, and for Lenny in particular, the use of alternative or complementary or integrative therapies has made us better able to treat him more effectively with traditional medicines. It's part of a whole treatment for him. Neither one by itself would have been sufficient, but together the sum is much better than the individual parts would be alone.

BODY & SOUL: What was your experience with Lenny?

ANDERSON: We always learn so much from our patients. Every single patient teaches us if we're open to that lesson. In Lenny's case, there have been multiple lessons for me. Lenny is an advocate by vocation and what he has latched onto in this particular instance is complementary therapies. The reason he has, is that he himself experienced complementary therapies in several forms which have been extraordinarily helpful to him, and have just allowed him to do so much better than he otherwise would have without them. I was very ignorant of and unaware of many of the complementary therapies to which Lenny had been exposed, so, if you will, he was my teacher. He opened my eyes, and he is opening the eyes of many other physicians, healthcare providers, and medical institutions to the availability, the breadth and scope of complementary therapies, and their potential value to patients. I think it's fair to say that he's taught me many lessons in life, but one of them is clearly the awareness and potential that exists in complementary therapies.

I think that when patients get the news that they have a fatal cancer, there are basically two ways that patients respond. The first, which is an unfortunate one, is to feel sorry for oneself—let the disease take control of their lives. In that instance, what happens is that patients do poorly very quickly. If you will, if you basically give in to your disease, it's a self-fulfilling prophecy. I mentioned that first because I want to contrast it in spades to Lenny Zakim's approach to his illness. What he did in this context is what he does with everything else in life: he looked at all of the options that were available, explored the world in terms of treatments, became as educated as he could about the illness that he had, tried to do the right thing in terms of conventional therapy, explored other areas, and in particular for him, complementary therapies and the potential that they had. What I'm trying to say is that he went after life with a zeal and a zest that he has always had, and maybe even more so after he heard the news of this cancer.

I can cite for you numerous specific examples, but maybe I can just mention one. Lenny has had a project over the years called Team Harmony, where he's

TEACHER

"I was very ignorant and unaware of the complementary therapies to which Lenny had been exposed, so, if you will, he was my teacher."

brought together, I believe, 10,000 students from Massachusetts into one forum to meet with political and sports leaders to discuss drug abuse, violence, and to dispel notions of bigotry and hatred in the world—trying, if you will, just to make the world a better place, to start at the grassroots level, at the level of schoolchildren. This program has been more successful than ever with Lenny at the helm, in spite of Lenny having a fatal illness. As a result of his efforts, this program happened in Washington, D.C. this year for the first time, and it will happen also in New York City. My bet is that if Lenny has anything to say about it, it will become a national program. I will cite one other example. After his illness occurred, Lenny had just an outpouring of love and support from so many individuals, all of whom wanted to help him. Rather than having that support channeled specifically to help him as an individual, Lenny founded what's called affectionately the 'Lenny Fund'. I've had the privilege of being at the ceremonies at which grants are awarded under the aegis of the Lenny Fund, small grants to multiple community-based organizations that are speaking out against drug abuse, that are trying to educate the underprivileged, that are providing medical care or childcare to folks who couldn't have it, otherwise. In other words, Lenny has turned the tragic news of his illness into a new zeal and a new zest for life, not only for himself, but as a motivation to do more good things for others.

I think I would characterize Lenny as a profile in courage. He's used this as an opportunity to educate the world about complementary therapies. I think this is so critical because, as studies have shown, roughly three-quarters of patients, as we sit here today, are using some form of complementary therapy. Often the healthcare providers, whether they be the doctors or nurses or others involved, are not aware that they might be doing these treatments. There's not a sharing, there's a reluctance on the part of some patients at least, and perhaps it's justified, perhaps the fear is that it wouldn't be accepted by the healthcare providers.

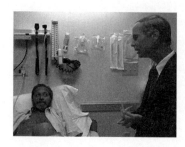 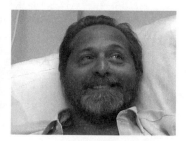 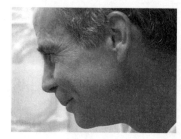

What needs to happen, and Lenny is really four-square behind this effort, is that there needs to be exposure to complementary therapies of many kinds. We need to explore their benefits, and in the same way as we do more traditional medicines, we need to evaluate the efficacy on the one hand, and the toxicity or side effects on the other, of some of the complementary therapies.

The reason I think this is so important is primarily the gain. Once we identify complementary therapies that we think work in a majority of patients or in a particular clinical setting, we need to get patients exposed to them so that they can do better in terms of their outcomes. A secondary benefit will be if certain complementary therapies are found to be adverse in the sense that they have side effects that wouldn't have been anticipated before, or even more importantly, if they have side effects that are related to the fact that they interact with some of the more traditional medicines that patients are receiving. We need to be aware of that, because in trying to do the right thing, it may be that some of the complementary therapies are interacting with the traditional therapies in an unanticipated adverse way that neither the patient nor the health-care provider currently knows. So as a result of Lenny's effort and many others, I think that some of these complementary therapies will be studied in a rigorous way, just as we do in other areas.

EXPOSURE

"There needs to be exposure to complementary therapies of many kinds. We need to explore their benefits, and in the same way as we do more traditional medicines, we need to evaluate the efficacy on the one hand, and the toxicity or side effects on the other."

MICHAEL LERNER

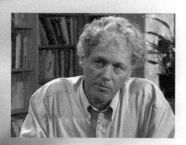

Michael Lerner, Ph.D., has become another important figure in Lenny's life since his cancer diagnosis. One of the country's leading authorities on complementary cancer treatments, Dr. Lerner is the president and founder of Commonweal, a health and environmental research institute in Bolinas, California, and co-founder of the Commonweal Cancer Help Program. He is the author of *Choices in Healing: Integrating the Best of Conventional and Complementary Approaches to Cancer.*

HARRIS: You met Lenny Zakim a while back when he came out to Commonweal. What was your sense of who he is as a person, his spiritual side, the issues that he's grappling with?

LERNER: I only spent a week with Lenny. I can't claim to know him well. But I believe that Lenny is—and I don't use these words lightly—I believe he's an authentic American hero. I believe that we live in a time where, if you watch the television or you read the newspapers, there aren't a lot of heroes around. And that children, and in fact all of us, need heroes at some level, people who are living from a deep place in themselves and are really making a contribution. My sense is that Lenny is making a contribution to social justice. He's making a contribution to human rights. He has dedicated his life to real racial dialogue, both in the United States and in getting Jews out of Russia and Eastern Europe, and in helping freedom in South Africa. Lenny has lived very, very fully. And now in the encounter with cancer, he has naturally embraced the rights and needs of cancer patients as part of what he is living for. So I was very profoundly moved by the week that I spent with Lenny. I've done about 90 of these week-long programs for people with cancer, the Commonweal Cancer Help Program, and often I have a sense that some of the people who come through are, in a very explicit sense, teachers for me. Lenny was one of those teachers. Lenny came to teach me some things.

HARRIS: Do you find that people like Lenny, who seem to have a real purpose to their lives, a real mission, do better over time?

LERNER: It depends on what we mean by that. I've seen some people who really do seem to live longer because they find that deep sense within themselves. But the other thing to remember is that cancer is a very difficult disease and that sometimes there is just a biological process that isn't going to be affected by anything that we do, or doesn't appear to be affected. I've certainly seen many people who are living from the deepest places within themselves in whom the progression of the disease seems quite inexorable. I think that it helps when it can help, and that often it is not able to help very much, in terms of life extension. But in terms of how we live, it helps profoundly.

HARRIS: One of the things that Lenny has found very helpful is this notion of imagery, but that's also controversial to some people, because they say, 'Well, wait a minute. If you're telling me that through the power of my mind I can make certain things happen, then the flip side of that is, it's my fault that I have this disease in the first place, because I've also made that happen.'

LERNER: Well, the Dalai Lama was once asked if people create their own diseases. And he simply laughed and said, 'People give themselves a lot of power when they say that, don't they?' The idea that we create our own diseases is, I think, a very unfortunate oversimplification of a very complicated process. I think that there are many origins of all diseases. What we're doing to the environment has a profound effect on our health. There's genetics; there's lifestyle; there's a wide range of things. The contribution that our psychology makes to our health is real, but it's very, very partial. But I think anyone who has a sense that they are responsible for a complex disease process just isn't looking at the totality of what's going on. Now, when it comes to people who say that the use of imagery is dangerous because it can make you feel guilty—because if you, through imagery, can shift the process of a disease, then you must also be held accountable for the disease—again, I think that is a very toxic oversimplification of the reality.

It's clear, there's evidence, that imagery can indeed shift some biological processes. That's true. There are some disease states where imagery can make an authentic difference in the process. That's true, too. But there is no good scientific evidence that imagery has a clear effect on cancer. There are many hypotheses about it, but there's no good scientific evidence about it. Nonetheless, the plausible aspect of it, that it might make a difference, that certainly it can affect quality of life and it might affect the biological process, is very real.

My more common experience with imagery is that people come in, and they've tried imaging healthy cells gobbling up cancer cells, and they can't do it. So they decide that they're no good at imagery. I always say to them, 'Well, before you decide you're no good at imagery, tell me, do you know how to worry? Because if you know how to worry, you're clearly good at imagery. Worrying is a very powerful form of imagery.' Then the only question is, 'Is the only imagery that you want to do in the course of this cancer worrying, or do you want to see if there are other ways that you can approach it?'

So I take a much broader perspective on imagery. To me, imagery is the language of the unconscious. Imagery is the language in which all the forces within us that we are not conscious of can speak to us. In that sense, it's not just about healthy cells gobbling up sick cells, it's all the intuitions and dreams and senses that we may have about where we should go forward in our lives right now. It's in that sense that paying attention to these is very important. You know, the Greeks knew this. They had the Aesculapian Temples of Healing. And the purpose of the temples was that people who were sick would come and sleep in these temples and await a dream of healing. When we have a life-threatening illness, there are all these unconscious forces that come very close to the surface and that are awaiting an opportunity to break through into consciousness. Imagery is simply one of the ways to elicit these unconscious forces and to listen to them, to see if they have wisdom for us about how to live.

HARRIS: It seems the point here is for the patient to get in touch with what's going on inside, that they may not have taken time to do before.

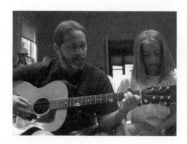
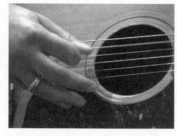
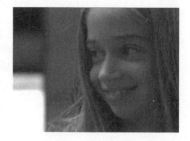

LERNER: That's right. Imagery is a word that we have for a wide range of ways to access healing sources of wisdom and compassion within us that we may not otherwise know about, and that have a tendency to rise and be ready when a life-threatening illness or a difficult time comes about. Accessing them through journals, through paintings, through dreams, through poetry, through meditation, accessing them is what it's all about.

HARRIS: Which is why some people describe it as a gift.

LERNER: I think it is a gift. I think, in a very literal sense, it's grace.

HARRIS: I want to ask you about the most significant categories of complementary, or perhaps unconventional, cancer treatments: the spiritual, the psychological, nutritional, physical, and then there's the traditional. Which have you found most helpful over time?

LERNER: I've studied complementary therapies for 15 years all over the world. I've studied hundreds of complementary therapies for cancer. In all that time, I've had four things that I've found have stood the test of time for me, in terms of findings. The first is, there is no clear-cut cure for cancer among the complementary cancer therapies. There is no cancer that clearly is cured by any complementary therapy. It's a very important thing to say, because that's why curative conventional therapies are the starting place for any reasonable person who has a curable cancer. The second is, there's very little scientific evidence on which to evaluate the much more interesting question, which is not whether there's a cure, because there isn't yet a clear-cut cure. The question is, do some people do better when they seek to integrate the best of conventional therapies and the best of complementary therapies in ways that make sense to them. The third is, that there is some scientific evidence, and strong anecdotal evidence, that many patients do better when they seek to integrate the best of conventional and complementary therapies. Clearly better in terms of quality of life, and potentially better in terms of survival or prevention of recurrence, as well. And the fourth finding is that while the fight continues in the trenches between the true believers in conventional therapies alone, who regard all complementary therapies as quackery, and the true believers in complementary therapies alone, who regard conventional therapies as a conspiracy against cancer patients of some kind—what's happened over the last 15 years is that at the top of the field, there's been this tremendous reaching out, this integration, a sense on everybody's part that none of us have all the answers for cancer. What we need to do is to help patients do what they want to do, which is not to give up conventional therapies, but to integrate the best of conventional and complementary therapies.

So, given that there's no clear-cut cure, how do we understand complementary cancer therapies? I developed a sort of an analysis of the main categories of complementary cancer therapies. I looked at them long and hard and I thought to myself, 'Well, there are spiritual approaches like prayer and laying on of hands, psychological approaches, support groups, psychotherapy, hypnotherapy, imagery, things like that. There are nutritional approaches, diet, nutritional supplements. There are physical approaches like yoga or Qi Gong or deep relaxation or exercise. There are traditional medicines, traditional Chinese medicine, Ayurvedic medicine, homeopathy, things like that. There are herbal approaches. There are pharmacological approaches. There are electromagnetic approaches. There are unconventional uses of conventional treatments, where people do conventional therapies but in unconventional ways. And, finally, there's a deep river that runs through the valley of complementary therapies, which is an emphasis on humane approaches to cancer. While not all complementary therapies deliver on that promise, most complementary therapies seek to be more humane. Those are 10 approaches.'

So then the question was, of those 10 approaches, how do you make choices? And as I looked at it, it seemed to me that if we took that list—spiritual, psychological, nutritional, physical, traditional medicines, herbal, electromagnetic, and so on and so forth—that the first four were qualitatively different from all the rest. And that the first four were different because anybody who begins to take care of themselves spiritually, psychologically, nutritionally, and physically, what happens to them? That's another way of asking the question in the more conventional sense. If you take care of yourself physically, mentally, emotionally, and spiritually, what happens to you? Naturally, other things being equal, you tend to become a healthier person. So if you have cancer, what happens to you? The truth is that, naturally, if there's time and space, you become a healthier person with cancer. Now what do the oncologists call a healthier person with cancer? They say that person has a better quality of life, which is obvious. And they also say that person has better what they call 'functional status.' Then you say to the oncologists, and I always say this to audiences of oncologists, 'Now tell me, what do your own research studies show about people who have better functional status with cancer?' The answer is that people with better functional status, in many cancers, tend to survive longer.

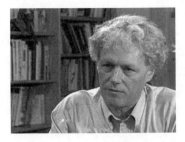
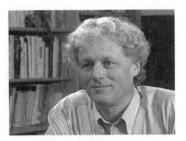

Now this, to me, is the authentic meeting place, right now, given the science, right now, between conventional and complementary therapies. We know that people with better functional status survive longer with many treatments for many cancers. It's not rocket science, because after all, if you're healthier, with a difficult disease and difficult treatments, wouldn't you think you'd do better? So if that's the case, then why shouldn't oncologists actively encourage patients who say, 'Doctor, I thought maybe a change in diet would help, or a support group would help.' Instead of dismissing that, why doesn't the oncologist say, 'You know, I'm so glad when a patient expresses an interest in these things, because it means I have a partner in this. It means that I am working with somebody who recognizes that this is a difficult disease, and the treatments are difficult, and wants to do something for himself. And so I want to encourage you in ways that make sense, to take care of yourself physically, mentally, emotionally, and spiritually. If I see you doing something that I think might be harmful to you, I'll tell you. I don't know a lot about complementary therapies, but I'm actively curious about what you are doing.' There's just a sense I have that if you took a thousand cancer patients, and half of them had an oncologist who dismissed all this, and the other half had an oncologist who responded this way, and we tracked them and saw what the outcomes were, I think that would be an interesting research project. But if I were among the people with cancer, I'd rather be with the group that has the oncologist who responded positively. I think it might work out better for them.

HARRIS: Which leads to the question, why don't more oncologists say exactly what you just did?

LERNER: Well, I think that's Lenny's life mission right now. I think Lenny is in the business of helping oncology rediscover its true calling as a healing process. Which, by the way, I believe many oncologists are profoundly committed to, themselves. But there is the other aspect of oncology that has forgotten that there is not only 'curing', but 'healing', and that that is recognized in the medical literature. They've forgotten that patients may take an active part in their own healing process. And I think Lenny's calling, right now, is to make a difference in this.

I make a fundamental distinction between healing and curing. Curing is what the physician seeks to offer you, and healing can only come from within ourselves. Healing is our province, as human beings. I think in any encounter with a disease, there's both the wonderful aspect of what science and biomedicine can bring, which are really one of the great creations of our civilization. But we have to remember that there's an ancient aspect of it that comes from within us, which is our response both to the disease and the treatments, and what we can bring to the table from that.

HARRIS: You've written, 'In a society that has forgotten how to meditate while healthy, many people are guided to a deep contemplation of the meaning of life only by illness.' It's a shame that it takes that.

LERNER: It is a shame. Yes, others have said that illness is the Western form of meditation, to say it very briefly. It takes place in a society that has lost the contemplative tradition to a large degree. But I think the good news is that the contemplative traditions are making a very powerful comeback throughout Western society. More and more people are finding that contemplation in all the traditions, in Judaism and Christianity and Islam and Buddhism and all the traditions, just has a very deep place in providing the reflective space that I think we all need to be aware of in our lives. Another thing that many of the wisdom traditions say is that most of us spend our lives asleep, that we go through life sort of sleepwalking, that everything is automatic. So anything that wakes us up is valuable, anything that reminds us and makes us present. Illness plays that role for many people. How often have you heard cancer patients say, 'This was a wake-up call'? Many people use it in that way.

HEALING

"I make a fundamental distinction between healing and curing. Curing is what the physician seeks to offer you, and healing can only come from within ourselves."

6 PARTNERS IN HEALING: MIND, BODY, AND PRAYER

I grew up in suburban Atlanta, "right smack dab in the middle" of the Bible Belt, as we say down home. Best known as the home of Lockheed Aircraft, Cobb County wasn't exactly rural in the mid-1960s, but it was not uncommon to see revival-meeting tents sprouting on vacant lots along the highway every spring, like mushrooms after the rain. Every church had the topic of that week's Sunday sermon posted prominently on a sign out on the front lawn, every high school had a chapter of the Fellowship of Christian Athletes, and the radio airwaves on Sunday morning were awash with preachers who spoke long and loud about hellfire and damnation.

It's fair to say that although I brought with me from childhood a vague belief in prayer as a mysterious and probably wonderful force, I never took the time to think very much about it during my 20s and 30s. I had a career to build; a marriage to sustain; a child to raise. As I rounded the bend into my forties, though, I began pondering the questions my Dad used to describe as "The Big Three": Who am I? Why am I here? Where am I going? Suddenly, spiritual issues of all kinds became more compelling.

Once I began a daily meditation practice five years ago, it was easier to acknowledge that there was some power greater than myself that could be tapped into at any time, whatever you might want to call it: God, Source Energy, Infinite Intelligence, All-That-Is. The spiritual part of me didn't need proof of any of that, but the skeptical journalist part of me did. As we began working on this series, then, it seemed like a good idea to investigate what science has to say about prayer and healing.

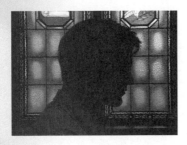

As you'll discover in this chapter, there are now a number of studies pointing the way toward something profound and powerful, although I'm not sure anyone can adequately describe it just yet. But when you hear what Dr. Larry Dossey has to say about scientific research on prayer and the mind/body connection, or why anesthesiologists believe that "healing statements" in the operating room can help people through surgery—well, it does make you wonder.

PEGGY HUDDLESTON

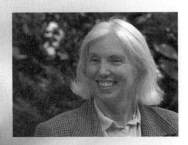 Peggy Huddleston is a psychologist in private practice in Cambridge, Massachusetts, and the author of *Prepare for Surgery, Heal Faster.* She is a principal investigator on the research project, "Patient-Centered Techniques to Enhance Surgical Outcomes," being conducted at three major Boston-area hospitals. Huddleston has a master's degree in theological studies from Harvard Divinity School.

HARRIS: How did this journey toward the concepts that you write about begin for you?

HUDDLESTON: It began when I was teaching workshops showing people what they can do emotionally and spiritually to speed their healing process. In a class of about 50 people, there would always be one or two who would raise their hand at the beginning of the class and say, 'I'm here because I'm having surgery in a couple of weeks. I'm giving my kidney to my sister.' Or, 'I'm having my thyroid out, and I'm scared. Is there anything I can do to reduce my fear?' They'd say, 'I can't sleep at night. My knees are shaking. And it gets worse the closer the surgery comes.' I just came up with five steps that seemed obvious that a person could use to, first, get very peaceful before surgery. So it was out of the context of seeing the need and being asked those questions.

HARRIS: How do you think the healing statements work?

HUDDLESTON: I think it's very simple. When a patient is unconscious with anesthesia, or even conscious and having a local anesthesia, in either state they're in a deep state of altered consciousness like hypnosis. So in that state when you say a statement like, 'Following this operation, you will heal very well and be very comfortable,' it's just like they're hypnotized and it goes straight in. After surgery, people report that they use, probably, 23 to 50 percent less pain

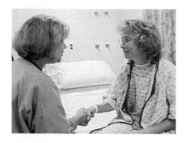
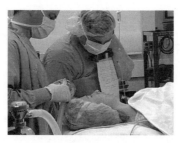
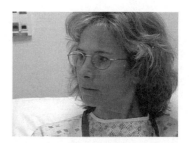

medication. That's what the research findings show, throughout this country and throughout the world.

HARRIS: So, basically, you're reminding your body to do what it already knows how to do?

HUDDLESTON: Yes, exactly. And then there's another statement that is read toward the end of surgery that actually lessens people's experience of nausea in the recovery room. Often people in the recovery room are throwing up and it's horrible, especially if you've got stitches in your stomach. It's the worst thing you want to have happen. So a very simple thing can be done. Just towards the end of surgery the anesthesiologist says, 'At the end of this operation you will be hungry for...' and the patient has filled in the name of their favorite light food, like strawberry yogurt or coffee ice cream. The anesthesiologist says that five times when the patient is still highly suggestible. So the patient in the recovery room wakes up hungry for strawberry ice cream, instead of having the nausea. The nausea was caused by the anesthesia. It's a foreign agent that the body is trying to get rid of, and normally it would get rid of it through the stomach. We don't know why it doesn't come out through the stomach now, but the stomach is saying, 'Oh boy, I want that strawberry ice cream.' And so there's very little, or usually no nausea. That's very, very unusual.

HARRIS: In terms of how patients respond to these ideas, how much of it is a feeling of relief that they can be in control, instead of surgery being exclusively something that is done to them.

HUDDLESTON: I think that's a large part of it, showing the patient there are concrete things they can do to participate in preparing for surgery, five specific steps they can use, so it gives them a sense of control where normally they'd feel helpless. And I think the other thing is, surgeons don't realize that patients are often frightened before surgery. Even if it's minor surgery, they're

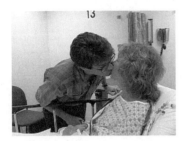 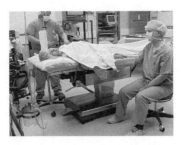 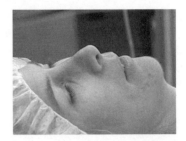

very, very scared. They can't sleep at night. I think it's because it's the closest we come to being dead. That's a pretty blunt way to say it, but there's a tremendous fear.

I find that fear will trigger unfinished emotional business. I kept seeing that happen with people I was working with, preparing for surgery. They'd come to me and say, 'I know I'm having a mastectomy and I know my crying is because of that, and it seems logical, but I am sobbing uncontrollably for hours and I can't stop.' So as I'd work with that patient, I'd discover that there was an earlier loss. There was one woman who, when she was 10 years old, her older brother had been killed in World War II and she'd been told not to grieve. The family all had a stiff upper lip, and they never saw their father cry. Her next great loss was her breast. That's a tremendous loss, and it triggered this earlier loss, this earlier grief that had never been grieved. She had to learn that's what that grief was, and I worked with her in feeling that grief and letting it release from her body. As people use the relaxation process they get very relaxed, so as a result, the emotions you've been stuffing down start to come to the surface, too. So it can be a very deep healing process for other wounds as a person is preparing for surgery.

C O N T R O L

"There are concrete things [patients] can do in preparing for surgery... so it gives them a sense of control, where normally they'd feel helpless."

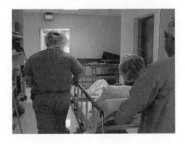

Alfred Daniels

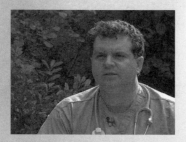

PROFILE

A staff anesthesiologist at New England Baptist Hospital in Boston, Alfred Daniels, M.D., has been reading healing statements to patients during surgery for several years now. He describes those who request these preparatory techniques as highly motivated individuals who are interested in decreasing complications and learning more about their surgical procedures, before they enter the hospital.

The healing statements he uses are tailored to the needs of the patient. "Frequently you're telling people that their tumor is all going to be removed, or that their joint is going to fit perfectly and last 25 years, instead of maybe the 15 it would have, otherwise. You're telling them they're going to be interested in doing physical therapy, which can be uncomfortable. It doesn't have to be specific to the type of surgery—anything related to thinking positive tends to help people. We have used healing statements such as, 'I am going to get up and walk tomorrow and feel comfortable.' It also seems to help people when they do their first therapy after surgery."

At first, says Dr. Daniels, he felt a little self-conscious, "because if you're whispering into someone's ear that's completely asleep, you gain the attention of the other people in the operating room. But most of the people in anesthesia are interested in educating people, especially if you're doing something that has very few side effects, such as talking to them or playing a tape. We're always interested if we can help someone that way."

One benefit of working with patients who have prepared for surgery ahead of time, according to Dr. Daniels, is that those individuals don't waste their energy on being afraid. Instead, they use their energy to help themselves. "Hospitals aren't the safest places in the world, basically, and everyone knows that. The food is not great. The bed is not great. They're noisy. There are a lot of problems with staying in hospitals. So if someone were motivated enough to get out of bed earlier and do their physical therapy earlier and leave earlier, it benefits everybody, especially the patient."

"If you're whispering into someone's ear that's completely asleep, you gain the attention of the other people in the operating room."

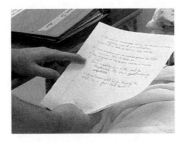 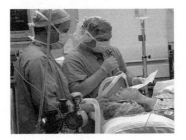 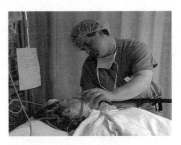

HARRIS: In some of the stories I've read about people who follow these techniques, they've said that not only did they come through the surgery just fine, but that basically it changed their life.

HUDDLESTON: I was so surprised when I'd hear people say, 'As I was lying on the gurney waiting for surgery outside the operating room, I felt more peaceful than I've ever felt in my life.' And I thought to myself, 'I don't think *I* would.' I began to ask them to tell me exactly what they were doing. Well, they were using the preparation steps exactly, and listening to a relaxation tape twice a day for usually about a week before surgery. People would call my office and say, 'I am so glad I'm having this operation.' I'd say, 'Why?' And they'd say, 'Because I was so frightened, I began to listen to that tape twice a day for the last week. I feel a peace and a love that I have never felt in my life, that I didn't know was possible to feel.' So, say they have two weeks before the operation. They're getting more and more connected to their own spiritual core as they prepare for surgery. That creates, in turn, the biochemistry of healing. It strengthens their immune system. We know from very good research that when a person gets relaxed, the number of their T-cells actually increase. The T-cells are those things that are made in our thymus gland that coordinate the entire immune system. When someone has AIDS, they're always looking to see what's the T-cell count. You want more instead of less. So we know that patients who are relaxed are enormously enhancing their immune function, which means they go into surgery with a strengthened immune function. They heal much faster. Most patients with major surgery leave the hospital a full day earlier, and they leave with this joy. They leave with a sense that they know how to participate in their healing—so they're very happy campers, which the surgeons also love.

LARRY DOSSEY

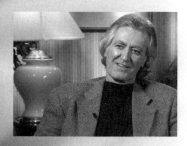

Larry Dossey, M.D., is one of the country's leading experts on spirituality and medicine. The former chief of staff at Humana Medical City Dallas in Texas and former co-chair of the Panel on Mind/Body Interventions for the National Center for Complementary and Alternative Medicine, he is currently the executive editor of the journal *Alternative Therapies.* Dr. Dossey is the author of *Healing Words, Prayer is Good Medicine, Meaning and Medicine,* and *Recovering the Soul.*

HARRIS: How did you, as a traditionally educated medical doctor, come to this notion that something like a healing statement read during surgery could be helpful, or that prayer could be useful in helping people heal?

DOSSEY: Well, I was blessed with a serious illness during my medical school career, indeed, back to the eighth grade. I had classical migraine headache. It was so severe, it even caused me to attempt to drop out of medical school at one point. I was afraid that I would harm someone in surgery, eventually. I thought that I should go into another line of work. It became obvious to me that my emotional life and my thoughts and my attitudes had a lot to do with this disability. When none of the medications or traditional approaches worked for me, I sought out a technique which was new on the scene in the late '60s and early '70s, called biofeedback. This is a way of hooking up to the electronic instruments and thinking in a certain way and using images and visualizations actually to change what your body is doing. This was a vivid demonstration to me that my own thoughts influenced dramatically what happened in my body. As I learned to develop this technique, the headaches virtually disappeared. Before this time I didn't even know I had a mind/body relationship; I was stuck in the old way of thinking that illness is only a reflection of what your body does to you. This was a great opportunity for me to learn about the impact of consciousness on the body, and this was a way in which I was able to use my own problems for insight, which is often the case. We talk about the 'wounded healer' tradition in medicine, which is using your own disabilities and problems to gain insights into the nature of healing.

HARRIS: You've written about a group called Spindrift which has conducted a number of experiments on the use of prayer. I wonder if you could explain a little bit about their work and what you think is going on there. This group does things like praying over beans and then finding that they grow faster.

DOSSEY: Well, they do grow faster. I was stunned by this work. It's good work. It's been replicated by many other researchers, but they were some of the first to do this. They designed a replicated system of interacting with non-human prayer subjects. They wanted to know if the effect of prayer on some-one was just a matter of positive thinking, or suggestion, or the old placebo response. And so they prayed, not for humans, for positive thinking could be a factor there, but for germinating seeds and growing plants and so on. They found in these controlled studies that the prayed-for seeds and plants actually germinated and grew faster. I was deeply impressed by this, because if plants and seeds respond to the effects of prayer, one can't say, 'Well, they were just thinking positively,' which has been the eternal, perennial, skeptical way of dis-posing of this sort of evidence. I went from looking at their experiments to scores of other experiments that had been done not only with seeds and plants, but with bacteria, the growth rates of fungi, the rate of healing wounds in rats and mice, for example. There are simply scores of very well-designed experi-ments out there that show, in ways that we can't completely explain as yet, that prayer has a positive effect on the state of the world and living organisms, not just human beings. So this is a great challenge, and a great opportunity, to bring the power of thought and intention and compassion and caring and love into the healing process. If you look at these studies, one of the things that is so dramatically apparent is the role of love and caring, because if the individual who is doing the praying in these experiments doesn't have this feeling of gen-uineness and compassion, these experiments don't work very well, and often they fall flat. I'm fascinated by that aspect of these studies, because this is in alignment with the perennial wisdom in the history of medicine that love is really important in what goes on between a doctor and a patient, which is the realization, I think, that we have almost forgotten in medicine. I think these studies in prayer and healing bring this out again. It's a lesson we desperately need to relearn.

HARRIS: Were you startled to find that there was scientific evidence about the value of prayer?

DOSSEY: I was shocked. I never heard of this. I considered myself a well-educated, modern physician. This simply wasn't part of my medical training, but there it was. And so the question was, what are you going to do with this? I have decided this is one of the best-kept secrets in modern medicine. Fortunately, it's becoming less of a secret. There are many schools in the country now that are responding to this information as it's being made public, and it's making a difference in how we educate young doctors. Three or four years ago, there were only three medical schools in the entire country that had courses devoted to exploring the role of prayer and healing, and the role of religious devotion in health. Currently, there are 40 medical schools which have courses like this, so I'm happy to say that there are academicians and scholars at our very best medical schools who are responding to this information or taking it on and incorporating it into medical school curriculums.

HARRIS: Once you came across these ideas, did that change how you practiced medicine?

DOSSEY: Not at first, because I had ingenious ways of weenie-ing out of engaging this information. I would say things like, 'Well, you know, this can't be important because I was never taught this. This can't be relevant to what I do as a doctor.' But something happens the more you engage this evidence. It becomes real to you, and I got to the point where I said, 'You call yourself a scientific physician. This looks like legitimate science. So are you going to let this make a difference in how you treat your patients?' At that time in my life, that made me very uncomfortable. I wouldn't have prayed for my own patients on a bet, because I didn't think it did anything. But I decided that I couldn't ignore the data, the evidence, any longer, so I reoriented my medical day. I

E X P E R I M E N T S

"There are simply scores of very well-designed experiments out there that show, in ways that we can't completely explain as yet, that prayer has a positive effect on the state of the world and living organisms, not just human beings."

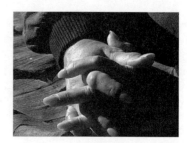

would go into my office earlier every morning and have my own prayer ritual, where I would actually pray for my patients that I'd be seeing in the hospital that morning, or who would be coming to my office that day. I maintained this prayer ritual for my patients until I chose to leave my practice a few years back.

HARRIS: Do you think it made a difference?

DOSSEY: One doesn't do randomized prospective studies in your own practice to see if it makes a difference, but I'm satisfied that it did, because of the studies, which I knew about at the time and which have since come forward, showing that prayer does make a difference.

HARRIS: And even if it didn't, I wonder if—did it make you feel better as a healer?

DOSSEY: Well, I think not only did it make me feel better, but I'm convinced it made my patients feel better as well, knowing that their own physician would go to the trouble of praying for them. Physicians are expected, rightly, to be technically competent, but going that extra mile and doing something like praying for your patients is really meaningful to patients. Studies have shown that this is what patients want their doctors to do. There was a recent study of patients who were hospitalized and the researchers asked them: 'Do you think your physician should be concerned about your spiritual life?' And 75 percent of these patients said, 'Of course. This is my doctor's business. She should be concerned about my spiritual life.' And 50 percent of the patients said not only that they wanted their doctor to pray *for* them, they wanted their physician to pray *with* them. So you see, this is a matter of intellectual indigestion mainly for doctors. Patients don't have any trouble with this at all. This is what they want. I think one of the reasons is that medicine has become so cold and remote and technical and so divorced from human feeling, that patients are hungry for a return of these qualities to healing. If you can bring the need for this together with good empirical science which shows that it's valuable, that it really does have a healing effect, we have no defense any longer for not doing this.

HARRIS: It makes you wonder if the old-fashioned country doctor was, in some ways, helping heal people by his presence, by the comfort of his concern.

DOSSEY: The way we talked about the old country doctor gives a clue about how we have put down these things in the past. We say he just used bedside

Robert Hunt

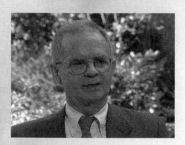

PROFILE

Robert Hunt, M.D., has been a gynecological surgeon in Boston for more than 30 years. Three years ago, after reading about Peggy Huddleston's techniques for relaxing before surgery, he started placing copies of her book in his office waiting room for patients to see.

"I think it's very difficult for older doctors and surgeons, sometimes, to make the transition to involve patients more in preparing for their surgery, using the techniques taught in Peggy's book. I was reluctant myself," recalls Dr. Hunt. "But then I began to realize that not only were the patients happier, it made my life a lot easier. The patients do better and require less time in the hospital, as long as you support what they're doing."

As for how and why the healing statements seem to work for surgical patients, "I think it just turns the healing process on," suggests Dr. Hunt. "I think it's nothing new to the body; the body knows this. We're the slow learners. I think once you can get an environment for positive influences to kick in on the patient's part, it happens. It's very natural."

Another major step for Dr. Hunt, personally, was realizing that a patient's outcome wasn't entirely up to his skill as a surgeon. "I'm just one part of the show. I'm not the show. I'm a participant. The nurses, the family, everybody. We're all part of a process circled around that patient to get her through whatever she's going to have done, and with a good result we get her back into her environment in good shape. It's been a learning process for me, about myself. And, I think, a very positive one, too."

The preparation techniques have also made a difference in how Dr. Hunt interacts with his patients in the moments before the surgery begins. These days, he takes the time to stand beside the operating table, the patient's hand clasped in his, as the anesthesiologist goes to work. "The funny thing is, after the post-op visit, they don't remember all the high-tech stuff. All they remember is, 'You held my hand, didn't you?' They remember that. And I'm so amazed. That's the one thing they remember."

"I think it just turns the healing process on...It's nothing new to the body; the body knows this. We're the slow learners."

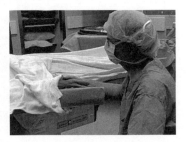 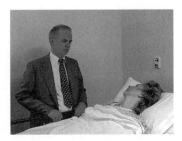

For this physician and surgeon, there is a compelling bottom line: preparation techniques prior to surgery, and healing statements read during the operation, do seem to make a difference in how well and how quickly his patients recover. "It works, and it makes my life easier, and I end up with a happier patient. I don't know what more I can hope for than that. If I could do that for the rest of my life, I will always have a smile."

manner, or how about all he did was use care and compassion, that this was just caring and empathy, or just the power of suggestion. We ought to get rid of the word 'just.' These are powerful forces. How do we know that? We can put them to the test in laboratory situations, and we can show the healing force and the healing power of compassion and empathy and love and caring.

HARRIS: How do you do that, though? How do you prove something like the notion that love heals?

DOSSEY: Well, you can do experiments where you instruct the person having the responsibility to do the praying, to do this in a cold, remote, unfeeling, uncaring way. This is what we call mimic prayer or mimic healing. It looks like the real thing, but the person doing it makes a conscious voluntary effort not to feel anything. Or, you can bring skeptics into the situation. You can say, 'Okay, you're going to be the healer.' They don't believe in it. It's not real for them. And when you use these kinds of subjects, the experiments don't work very well at all. On the other hand, if you bring legitimate and authentic people who deeply believe in the power of love and compassion and empathy, then you see these dramatic effects in the laboratory. So you can assess this. The experimenters have something available to them called empathy rating scales.

You can ask them the extent to which you felt love and compassion during the experiment. I'll grant you we don't have any love meters which you can plug into people and get a direct readout of the presence of love, but we can do a pretty good job of assessing it.

HARRIS: Is it important to have scientific evidence for some of these ideas?

DOSSEY: I think most people who are sick and go to a doctor could care less about whether or not love is documented scientifically to have an effect. It just feels right for most people, and that's the end of the discussion. But if we want to have an effect in the way that medicine, scientific medicine, is practiced in our culture, we better go through science if we can. Whether anyone likes it or not, science is one of the most powerful forces in our culture, and if we can bring science to bear on these issues, I think we're obliged to do that. If we want to make a difference culturally and professionally, we need to bring science into the bargain. I think also it's important to bring science in because it's just a fact of life that we do have a logical, rational side to us, and we need to try to bring together analytical, intellectual faculties together with intuitive and spiritual ways of looking at things. If we don't do that, we're going to be living a divided, schizophrenic sort of life, and this is pathological. This is what we've done in this culture and in Western cultures in general for over 100 years. This is an unhealthy way for human beings to try to live, to partition our lives into two separate, indivisible parts. If we can bring science into the mix, and we can ally it with our spiritual and intuitive qualities of thinking and being, we're going to be healthier human beings as a result.

HARRIS: You've written about something that you describe as 'Era One', 'Era Two' and 'Era Three' medicine. What is the difference between those three?

DOSSEY: This is a way of thinking about the evolution of medicine since it first became scientific in about the mid-1800s. Era One, really, is mechanical

L O V E

"Love is really important in what goes on between a doctor and a patient, which is the realization, I think, that we have almost forgotten in medicine. I think these studies in prayer and healing bring this out again. It's a lesson we desperately need to relearn."

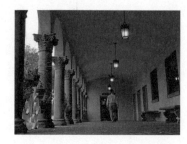

medicine. It's drugs, surgical procedures, treating the body as a machine. Era Two began in the 1950s, thereabout, and today we call this the mind/body approach. This was the realization that people's minds and thoughts and emotions could affect their own body. Era Three goes farther. That's the era that's opening up today. Era Three suggests that not only can your mind affect *your* body—your thoughts and intentions and prayers and attitudes can even affect *my* body. This is manifested in the experiments on distant prayer, distant healing, sometimes called distant intentionality, the evidence for which is utterly compelling, so Era Three is the latest vision in how consciousness gets in on the active healing process.

HARRIS: Let's talk a little bit about this notion of distant prayer, or being able to send thoughts to somebody else. There is a Princeton University study that you cite about this—what was that all about? And, also, how are we to think about the possibility of actually 'sending' thoughts to someone else?

DOSSEY: I think we're going to think about sending thoughts to other people at a distance with great difficulty until we get used to it. This is a mind-boggling idea for a lot of people who stumbled onto this area for the first time. But the data isn't going to go away. The Princeton data is only one of scores of studies which have replicated the ability of people to send thoughts to other people at a distance. Just to be very brief about this: at the Princeton laboratories, the Princeton Engineering Anomaly Research Laboratory, a computer will select an image and it will be given to someone on site at Princeton, who will look at it and try to convey mentally the contents to someone who is a long way off. This person may be on the other side of the earth. But at a given moment the receiver of this information registers it, writes it down, describes it, and then this information is fed back into a computer, which decides whether or not there's a hit or a miss between what was sent and what was received. There have been over 300 of these experiments done at Princeton alone, and in many instances the information gets through in camera-like, accurate detail. But I find most stunning the fact that in the majority of these instances, the receiver gets the information up to *three days* before it's even sent. Now, this is an outrageous possibility for people who believe that this is just not possible. But the data speaks for itself.

How should we think about this? If we want to engage this information, we're going to have to rethink the nature of the consciousness of our mind. I think we're going to be pushed to a new way of thinking about consciousness, which says this: there are some qualities of who we are, some aspect of our mind that is not limited or localized or confined to the brain and the body and maybe not even to the present moment. It's what we call non-local. It's beyond space. It's beyond time. It's what Dr. David Chalmers calls fundamental in the universe, perhaps on a par with matter and energy. It's everywhere. So, you see, the idea that we're sending information to somebody may be a wrong way to think about this. There may be no place for consciousness to 'go.' It may already be everywhere. If we're able to think in these new ways, I think these ideas, these experimental findings can seem a lot less outrageous to us. It would be shocking if our ideas of the mind stayed the same. Ideas evolve in medicine and in science. So it's not a question of whether or not there are images of what the mind happens to be or whether it's going to evolve. These images will change. We know that. The question is: what's the new picture going to be?

The new picture is going to be one in which we allow the mind to escape being confined to the brain and body. If we're willing to do that, then we'll be in a position of honoring this new challenging data, which comes not just from these studies at Princeton but in the studies in medicine, in distant intercessory prayer. I think it's urgent that we open up to these new views of consciousness. If we do not, we're going to find ourselves in the awkward position of having to deny actual scientific evidence for what the mind does. This will be tragic, because it will amputate some very powerful tools we have available in healing. Medicine desperately needs these new ideas of consciousness. Without them, healing will be much less effective.

HARRIS: Let's say you're right. What does that mean for health care, if your active prayer for Aunt Sally out in California when you're on the East Coast makes a difference. What does that mean about how health care is likely to change in the next 20, 30, 50 years?

DOSSEY: There are two aspects I would bring out about the implications. One is that if our consciousness can make a difference at a distance, for example through distant prayer, that means that health care is not just an individual effort. If you're sick, I can help you. And if I'm sick, you can help me. Health care can become a collaboration, a mutual effort. It doesn't just depend on what you decide to do about your health. The other thing is this—and I think this is the most exciting implication of all—if there's some aspect of our mind, as these studies suggest, that is truly outside of space and time, completely unlimited in time, then something about us is immortal and eternal. It's completely free from time. We've had a concept in the history of the West that honored this realization. We used to call that quality of consciousness, the soul. And it's not an exaggeration to say that these studies point like an arrow to the old idea of the soul, of immortality. One of the goals of modern medicine has been to help people live a long time. I think one of the implications of this data is that there is some aspect of who we are that is already immortal and eternal. Why? Because it's outside of time. I call this realization 'eternity medicine', in contrast to the temporal, time-based medicine that dominates our thinking today. I can't think of a more majestic thing than for a doctor to be able to tell a sick patient, 'Look, we're going to do all we can in this situation. But let's suppose we fail, and you die. You're just going to have to settle for immortality.' I think that's a pretty good thing to be able to tell a patient.

HARRIS: How is it, do you think, that we've gotten to the place where even talking about matters like the soul or immortality—it puts people off a little bit. They may want to hear it, but they feel a little awkward about it, too.

DOSSEY: There has been a gradual divorce of spiritual and religious thinking from science for well over 150 years. The most dramatic split came over the theory of evolution, the great Darwinian debate when religion and science really came to blows in the Western cultures. Since that time we've developed this schizophrenic way of thinking that these things are totally opposed to each other, that they cannot be harmonized and reconciled. I think this has had a deadening effect on people's sensibilities. It isn't written in stone that you can't get spirituality and science together. We made that up. That's a cultural assumption, and we're in the happy position now of being able to bring these things together. I predict that is what is going to happen, and we will look back at this

SCIENCE

"I think most people who are sick and go to a doctor could care less about whether or not love is documented scientifically to have an effect. It just feels right for most people and that's the end of the discussion. But if we want to have an effect on the way that medicine is practiced in our culture, we better go through science if we can."

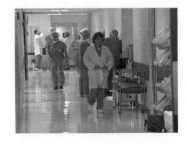

Tommie Sue Montgomery

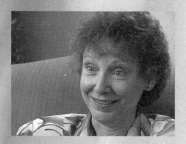

LIFE

A former professor of political science at Agnes Scott College in Atlanta, Tommie Sue Montgomery is among a number of patients who have used relaxation techniques to prepare for surgery. When she was first told that her kidney problem had developed to the point that surgery was going to be necessary, "my initial reaction wasn't terror as much as it was something crashing down on me that I didn't need at that point in my life. This couldn't have come at a worse time—I was unemployed and looking for a job, a long-term relationship had just ended, and now this happened on top of it." In addition to the usual fears patients may experience prior to an operation, Tommie Sue also had to overcome bad memories of a surgical experience 18 years earlier.

While waiting for a CAT scan shortly after her diagnosis, Tommie Sue discovered *Prepare for Surgery, Heal Faster*, in the hospital gift shop. She sat down and began to read, and finished the book before she went to bed that night. A few days later, she called to order the relaxation tape that accompanies the book.

Does it work? "Oh boy, does it ever. The more you listen to it, the more adept you become at relaxing," she laughed. "I listened to it last night, 36 hours before my surgery, and I was fairly tense. But by the time the tape was over, I was almost asleep."

Tommie Sue began keeping a journal of her thoughts and feelings prior to surgery. In early July, just five days after she read Huddleston's book, she wrote, "Peggy Huddleston, you've unleashed Scarlett O'Hara. It's all set. I'm going to be unconscious for two-and-a-half hours. They're going to cut me open and sew me up with a tube hanging out my side. But I absolutely believe it is going to be okay. I continue to feel positive and most important, in control. Now I just need to learn to relax on command!"

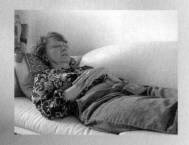
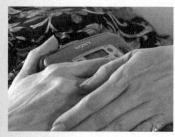
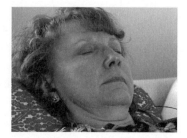

We checked in with her again shortly after her operation. By the morning of her surgery, Tommie Sue told us, her new relaxation techniques were still working well. A pre-operative check showed that her blood pressure was normal, her anxiety under control. She was so unconcerned, in fact, that she sat in the surgical waiting room doing needlepoint as she awaited the arrival of the anesthesiologist.

Four weeks later, a delighted Tommie Sue reported, "My recovery has been far better than I had any right to expect, although I certainly prepared for precisely this kind of outcome. I have to say that I never really experienced pain. The healing statements that I had prepared for use in surgery, as well as the healing imagery that I had used before—both, I think, contributed significantly to my recovery, as well as the extraordinary support group of friends, both in the community and in my church."

How did this experience compare with her surgery 18 years ago? "It was all the difference in the world, because the first time I didn't know what to expect and I was absolutely terrified. This time I was comfortable, and I've healed extraordinarily well."

"I have to say that I never really experienced pain. The healing statements that I had prepared for use in surgery, as well as the healing imagery that I had used before—both, I think, contributed significantly to my recovery."

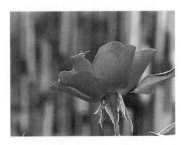
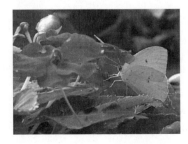
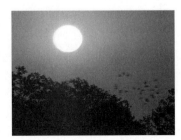

historic period and say, 'How did we get it so wrong?' I think that this divorce between science and spirituality is phony. It is one of the causes of more pain and suffering and anguish for so many people. We simply can't calculate it. So this is one of the great cultural healings that needs to happen in contemporary society, and, fortunately, I think we can see where this is headed. We are bringing it back together. I think most people, including an increasing number of scientists and doctors, would say it's about time.

HARRIS: We were speaking of the scientific evidence about prayer a minute ago. From the data you've seen, is there a 'right' way to pray?

DOSSEY: People have been looking for that right way to pray since time immemorial and nobody's come up with it. You can't certainly find the right way to pray in any of these studies, because people pray in a variety of ways. I love this result. I have some friends in the religious community, however, who are horrified by it, because they think that there surely must be some better ways to pray than other ways. Unfortunately for them, but fortunately, I think, for most folks, we can say that nobody's cornered the market on prayer. Nobody has identified one way that just sort of knocks all the other ways cold. This is important for our time because this democratizes and universalizes prayer. It says that prayer is an activity for which there is no formula. It belongs not to specific religions and techniques and strategies but to the entire human race. One can show that love and genuineness, compassion and authenticity, feeling it in the heart, is probably the most important factor of all. How this is sliced and diced in terms of religious outlook is very arbitrary. This says something about tolerating difference in spirituality and religious devotion. We can show that the prayers in experiments of born-again Christians are effective. We can show also that you bring in Buddhists and have them pray, and Buddhist prayer works just fine. Buddhism is not even a theistic religion. Buddhists don't pray to the idea of a personal God. This would horrify a lot of people in our culture, that Buddhist prayer, which is not theistic, can be answered. But there you have it. You do the experiments. You see that both types of prayer work. That is a result about which I'm joyful.

IDEAS

"Medicine desperately needs these new ideas of conscious-ness. Without them, healing will be much less effective."

HARRIS: In speaking about the value of prayer, it occurs to me that when something happens to someone you love—let's say, they're so sick they land in the hospital—often we feel so helpless, as if there's nothing we can do for them. What you're suggesting is that there's something very powerful we can do for them, and that you don't have to be a medical doctor to do it.

DOSSEY: That's correct. One can always extend empathy and caring and compassion and love. Sometimes we wrap that up into something we call prayer. There is an intervention that's always available. We don't have to let the doctor do everything. That's not to say that the disease will always go away—and we shouldn't trivialize prayer because the prayer isn't answered the way we want it to be—but there's always a sense in which prayer does work. If we can allow it, it can always help us bridge a sense of something greater, a sense of something richer and deeper and wiser than our individual self. That can always be healing, in a certain sense. It may not always be curing in the sense of making a disease go away. Everyone is going to die. No matter how majestic our therapies become, no matter how powerful our prayers are, the statistics are pretty powerful. The statistics are suggestive that no one is going to escape physical death. One of the promises of prayer is, there is some aspect of who we are that's beyond space and time, that's immortal and eternal, and it's highly therapeutic for people to be able to get in touch with that. It's particularly consoling during moments when we're facing death, or a loved one is facing death. When you compare that with the findings that diseases do have a way of responding positively to that kind of impact, then we should be using this in medicine. We should make a place for this.

HARRIS: Can you give me some specifics about studies in which the evidence was absolutely overwhelming that someone praying *here* for someone else over *there*, that it really worked or that it really helped?

DOSSEY: Probably the most sensational study on prayer this century was published in 1988. It came out of San Francisco General Hospital. It was a study of patients with heart attacks or severe chest pain that was done by a cardiologist, Dr. Randolph Byrd. Dr. Byrd took 393 patients who were in the coronary care unit at San Francisco General Hospital, and half of these people were prayed for and half were not. Everybody, however, received state-of-the-art, high-tech medical care for the problem. To make a long story short, the prayed-for group did better on many accounts: they needed less potent medication, they had fewer complications. Also, nobody in the prayed-for group had to have a tube put down the throat and be hooked up to the mechanical ventilator, while 12 people not receiving prayer had to have that done. The people receiving prayer had a lower instance for the need for CPR, cardiopulmonary resuscitation, than the people not receiving prayer. I think most physicians would look at this study and say if you had to choose which group you'd want your patient to be in, you'd put them in the prayed-for group. And probably it's the case that if what was being evaluated had not been prayer but a new medication, we really would have called this a therapeutic breakthrough. That study did grab headlines when it was published. I think, though, that we ought to hang onto our hats because that was just a teaser.

There are many other studies in progress. One that has particularly grabbed my attention was just completed at California Pacific Medical Center by Dr. Elizabeth Targ. This was a study in patients with advanced AIDS. These patients were divided into two groups. They all received comparable treatment technically, medically, but half the people, unknown to them, had their names assigned to distant healers, people who used various techniques, all of which were based on empathy and compassion and, frequently, prayer. The people who received the prayer had a much better outcome. They had a higher quality of life. Fewer of them died. Again, these studies were not subtle. These were dramatic differences. You look at these studies and you think, this is something that anyone in their right mind ought to be using. It saves lives. It makes people healthier in the process. In any other context we'd just call that good medicine. This would be a valuable intervention. But still we occasionally see people getting their backs up over this and thinking this is somehow illegitimate, because it smacks of spirituality and religion. I think we ought to be covering our bases and using anything that works, whether or not we call it drugs, surgical procedure or spiritual intervention.

HARRIS: We've been talking a lot about the evidence that prayer can be helpful. Do you have any evidence or any theories about *how* it works? Is this the patient's own belief system kicking in which is helping them get better? Or is this something else?

DOSSEY: All of the above. I think we know enough now about how healing works to say that the patient's belief system is important. It probably does make a difference whether, as we used to say, the person has faith. But that's not the only thing. There are powerful studies which show that faith doesn't have to be present for prayer to work. How do we know that? Well, these are what we call double-blind studies. For one thing, in many of these studies the patients don't even know they're receiving the prayer at the time they're getting it. But more importantly, many of these studies have been done not with humans where positive thinking and faith can play a role, obviously, but with non-humans. For example, you can take tissue from human beings. You can take red blood cells, which has been done in one particular experiment. You can ask or pray or intend or wish or want them to behave in a certain way and they do. These are fanatically precise, controlled double-blind studies. Red blood cells don't think positively. They don't have placebo responses. They aren't subject to suggestion and expectation as whole human beings are. So if the prayer works on red blood cells, you can say that this goes beyond positive thinking. More outrageously, you can pray that these five test tubes of bacteria will grow faster than these five, which are the controls, and statistically, in experiment after experiment, they do. This is powerful evidence that whatever role faith may play in human beings, it's not absolutely necessary for this effect to happen. So in actual practice, a lot of things go into the effect: there's a role for faith and expectation and positive thinking, but there's also a role for prayer or intentions that go beyond the power of positive thinking and faith.

HARRIS: You've also suggested that maybe it's a good thing that not all prayers get answered. Why not?

DOSSEY: Well, I think that there are some pretty nasty prayers out there, and it's a blessing in disguise that they are not always answered. I used to think that prayer was universally a wonderful thing, and I think most people in our culture sort of believe that. There are side effects to prayer just like there are side effects to any known medication or surgical procedure, and some people realize this. I was stunned in 1994 to discover a Gallup poll which found that five percent of American people actually prayed for harm for other people. Now that's just the one in 20 who will own up to it. If you do the numbers, that's over 10 million Americans out there praying for harm for other people. If we had 10 million Americans who were sick with any disease, we'd call that an epidemic. There's an epidemic of negative praying going on in our country, and any right-thinking individual ought to ask, does that do anything? Interestingly, you can take this into the laboratory, and although you can't test negative prayer on humans because that's illegal—you can't do a study designed to harm people—you can test the effects of negative thoughts and intentions and prayers and wishes on those bacteria in test tubes, and you can inhibit their growth, compared to controls, with negative thoughts and intentions and prayers. There is a negative, inhibitory effect. And I think that we ought to give more thought to the effect that negative thoughts and wishes and emotions have on those people to whom we intend them. I think there's a tremendous amount of negative thinking going on in our culture. I think we would be blind not to acknowledge this. We just sort of dismiss this in many different ways. Freedom of expression, the role of the media, and so on. But there's an ethical dimension of thinking that we have not yet come to terms with. I think all the negativity gets around. And I think there's evidence in the laboratory that we ought to seriously consider the negative consequences of our thoughts, wishes, intentions, and prayers.

HARRIS: I want to read something that you've written: 'Science and spirituality can now stand side by side in a complementary way with neither trying to usurp or eliminate the other.' What do you mean by that?

DOSSEY: We've had this titanic struggle where science and religion have been trying to duke it out now, one dominating the other, for well over 150 years. I have felt the pain that this causes, this split between science and spirituality, personally. I think when we send our kids off to college they experience that, because the message that we give people who enter science is, 'Look, you have two ways of living your life. You can choose to be spiritual and religious and intuitive and flaky, or you can be intellectual and rational and logical and scientific.' So you've got to choose in your life. When we dispatch our kids to colleges and universities they get this message in spades. I think it's a damaging message to give anyone, particularly young children who are trying to make sense of the world. How should they live their life? Because this forces a division in the human psyche that is unnatural. We have both an intellectual and a spiritual side. To tease them apart makes no sense, and it causes immense pain. I think that we face a great challenge in bringing these together. The former French Minister of Culture and great novelist, Andre Malraux, said once that the 21st century will be spiritual or it will not be at all. This for me captures the urgency of the situation. We desperately need to bring together science and spirituality. Our future as a species may depend on it.

HARRIS: Is science open to that idea?

DOSSEY: There's a stereotypical piece of nonsense which needs to be laid to rest, the idea that all scientists are agnostics and the best scientists are atheists. This isn't true. There is a study which was published in April of 1997 in which American biologists, physicists, and mathematicians were asked about their spiritual views. Forty percent of these scientists said, yes, they do believe in a Supreme Being, and more than that they believe in the form of a Supreme Being that would respond to distant, intercessory prayer. Well, this dismisses this idea that science is just a purely godless pursuit that has no spiritually redeeming qualities whatsoever. And, unfortunately, this is the image that so many people have of science. I think within science there is this quality which is not recognized, that is deeply spiritual. I think, and I trust and hope, that the evidence that prayer does have effects in medicine and in healing will encourage a lot more scientists to come forward and to own up and claim the spiritual urges that they deeply sense.

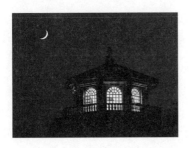

7. MAKING WORK MEANINGFUL

My father always said that the ideal job was one that you liked so much, you would be willing to do the work even if you didn't get paid for it. Now, many people might read those words and snort indignantly, "Oh, yeah? And what about paying the bills, and putting food on the table, and…"

Well, yes. There is that. But there is value in his rosily optimistic view of the work world. With our jobs occupying so many hours of our day, doesn't it make sense to try to find something that fills those hours in a satisfying way? As poet David Whyte points out in the next chapter, when we spend our time engaged in work that feels like drudgery, solely to support ourselves or our families, eventually we will get angry at the very people we say we love. If we feel that their demands are keeping us shackled to work that brings us no pleasure, eventually we will resent those who seem to be forcing us to do it.

Redefining work as something that is satisfying and pleasurable may be a fairly radical notion, the sort of thing that is only possible in a rich country with a vibrant economy. "There are two ways to be rich," I remember reading once. "One is to have a lot of money. The other is to want less." But it seems to me that wanting *less* is not the answer, as much as wanting *differently*. Wanting more time, instead of a more expensive car or bigger home. Wanting more freedom and flexibility, instead of a vacation we can't afford. Wanting to feel more in control of what we do and when, instead of being at the mercy of a demanding boss who has little concern for the deeper issues of our lives.

I personally believe that we can have anything we want, as long as we want it badly enough. The struggle is to figure out exactly what that is, so that we can set about pursuing it. Life is too short to spend our days being miserable. For each of us, I suspect, there is some special task that we can perform very well—maybe even better than anyone else in the world. How will you know when you've found it? Because it won't feel like work. Your heart will sing and you'll fling back the covers each morning, eager to get on with that day's assignment, whatever it might be. Your entire being will be filled with the knowledge that you are doing exactly what you want to be doing at this moment in time. Oh, yes. You'll know. And both your body and mind will thank you for it.

DAVID WHYTE

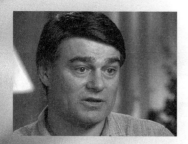

Poet David Whyte uses his perspective on creativity to work with many American and international companies as a consultant in the field of organizational development. His books of poetry include *House of Belonging*. He is also the author of *The Heart Aroused: Poetry and the Preservation of the Soul in Corporate America.*

HARRIS: I want to start with the notion of poetry and corporate life coexisting. I think in the minds of many people those two are not only not neighbors, they are not even in the same zip code. Can they be?

WHYTE: I think they have to be, because we spend so much of our waking lives in the workplace. When you think about it, we spend more time in the workplace than we do with our nearest and dearest. It's quite sobering to total up the time you spend at work against the time you spend with your family. I'm speaking now of time when you're awake and not simply asleep in the same house. We spend more time in the workplace than we do in our places of worship. We spend more time in the workplace than we do in the natural world. If we're not asking questions that are germane to what it means to be fully human in that workplace, what we're saying is, I will only ask the real questions about what I'm about, and the nature of my belonging to this amazing creation, in about 10 percent of the time that is left to me. But what happens is that when people get to that 10 percent of time, they're actually so exhausted that they can't bring anything real to it.

My question is, how do you bring these two worlds of poetry and business together? It's a question that not only has a kind of personal pressure behind it, there are also very good business reasons for doing that. Almost every company that has any kind of creative pizzazz about it is asking for more creativity from its people—for more adaptability, for more vitality. They're asking people to go the extra mile. Those qualities of adaptability and creativity, by the way, which are ancient qualities that we have all wanted for ourselves for thousands of years, can't be coerced. You can't legislate them. You can't say, 'Sarah, come into my office. I'd like an increase in the creativity quotient of 8.9 percent this week.' The request is absurd, because there's no switch inside me that I can get at where I can just turn that creativity on. If there was, I would have done it for myself years ago. What will get me into a place where I will want to be more creative, want to be more engaged, want to adapt, will be a situation in which I'm invited into the conversation—the conversation of what we're about in the workplace, what we're producing, what we're providing—and having a sense that there's something real there for me, that I'm seen and heard and my gifts are wanted in the world. That will create a situation where I'll want to give those gifts. And the conversation itself will surprise me into my own creativity.

HARRIS: When I first thought about talking with you about workplaces, I thought, 'Oh, good, here's someone who can talk about how workplaces can become more humane.' But, in fact, your approach is very much how the individual looks at work, and what he or she has to contribute, as well as how the organization functions.

WHYTE: Yes. I think it's the place to begin. Much of what we have to do to transform the workplace does not have to do with macro-massaging the system or with new strategies. We've reached the end of the road, as far as strategy is concerned, in getting to the conversation that produces creativity, produces a sense of community, belonging, and a sense of rightness about your work. The work of poetry is to give people the quality of courage, and a sense that what they're engaged in has very high stakes. You get this one life. You spend most of it in the workplace. If you do not have your deepest desires in sight—and it's interesting that the word desire comes from the old Latin, meaning 'of the

D A N G E R

"You get this one life. You spend most of it in the workplace. If you do not have your deepest desires in sight... you're in danger of losing everything that is precious to you, and living out a life that is like a shell."

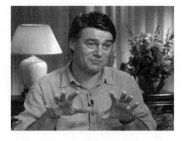

stars'—if you do not keep your star in sight, you're in danger of losing everything that is precious to you, and living out a life that is like a shell. You build a house for yourself, which you haunt like a ghost instead of inhabiting as a real person. In order to keep the house of your work real, you have to engage in conversation every day, just as you do in a family or a relationship.

HARRIS: You've written that, 'Work is drama and theater, the place where life unfolds to our tragic or comic satisfaction.' I'm wondering if that means that if you hate your work, to some measure, you hate your life.

WHYTE: I'd say so. Especially today where there's so much asked of people in the workplace. There are obviously times in anyone's life where you have to put bread on the table, and you'd be thankful for any work. But if there comes a time when you've gone beyond that, and you've told yourself that there's no other possibility except this one work, and you're actually giving yourself to it but in a way in which you're totally depleted, you do start to hate the rest of the world. More seriously, you start to hate the people close to you, too. You start holding them at emotional gunpoint to hand over all the qualities you should be trying to bring about yourself in your own life.

HARRIS: I imagine a certain amount of resentment might play a part here. 'How dare you be so ungrateful? I'm doing this for you. I'm throwing away my life for you...'

WHYTE: Exactly.

HARRIS: '...to put bread on the table.'

WHYTE: That awful hatred of your work becomes like a weapon pointed at the people close to you, especially at the people you're supporting. Responsibility becomes a burden, instead of people taking joy in providing. So there's a tremendous connection between the conversation we have at home, and the conversation we have in the workplace. If I am totally committed financially, then if I lose my work for even a month or so, and get off that hamster wheel which I'm on month by month, the whole financial edifice would come crashing to the ground. If that's the situation in my life, how much courage can I have around a meeting table? Very little. Whenever it gets near the point that my identity in that company is threatened, I will always finesse the conversation. I will have no courage, because I have allowed my home life to rob me of courage in my work life.

So both those conversations—of home life and work life—have to be brought together. I may have to say to my son, 'I've been telling you wrong all these years. I may not have been saying it out loud, but I've been telling you through my actions that if I provide all these material goods for you, you're going to be happy. It's not true. It hasn't been true for me, so why should it be true for you? You can't be looking to me for your next pair of inline skates. I need you to be more on my side because it's robbing me of my courage at work.' That's a difficult conversation for anyone.

We know how identities have a momentum of their own. We feel if we even break one part of it, the whole thing will break apart. That's the same fear we have about having a conversation that may change a system in our workplace. It's the same fear we have in beginning a conversation that may change our systems at home. What the poetic tradition is saying, again and again, is all you have to do is come out of hiding. You've got to find your own voice, no matter how mouse-like that is, and you have to begin the conversation. You begin it in whatever way you can, and when you've begun the conversation, you just stay there through it. The conversation itself will bring you to a new place.

This is what I think poetry grants us. Poetry is in such demand in the workplace. I have hundreds of poems memorized, my own and others. I work with these poems in a kind of extemporaneous way, to get into places and into conversations that we can't get into through our normal inherited workplace jargon. That jargon is not a language that's large enough for the kind of theater we find ourselves in now, in the new post-modern workplace, in the new office cubicle, in the new relationships between colleagues, or between boss and subordinate. All of those relationships are changing completely, and the world of work that we inherited from our parents is gone.

We have a world of work that is much more dependent on conversation, on relationship. It's one of the reasons why women, in a sense, are pre-adapted for this new post-modern workplace, because they have in their bodies the knowledge of the firsthand use of conversation. Men have to learn that more. Men have other virtues, but it's not in the area—at least as young men—of conversation. Young men are constantly surprised, for instance, in the beginning of a relationship or a marriage, that even though they had a conversation last week, they have to have it again this week. The hope in the young masculine psyche is that you can have one conversation at the beginning, and then coast for a good few years, at least, before there's another one. Of course, this is the whole inherited masculine model of the workplace—the hope that you can have systems in place that take care of everything, and therefore, you won't have to talk about it.

HARRIS: Ever again.

WHYTE: Exactly. One of the great impacts of the new work world is on the masculine identity. Some men are adapting to it, and some men are just having terrific pain and difficulty with it. You can say the same things for certain organizations. Some are adapting well to it. Some don't know what to do at all. They can't get there from here. They need a completely new language. And I think it's the language, which is so rich in our literate English traditions, that can help us form new conversations, to have the conversations that will help us change.

Like every man, I've had difficulty with conversation in my life. But there was a tremendous moment where I suddenly realized that I didn't need to do all the work of conversation—that the conversation itself can carry the burden of change. It was the first time I ever went kayaking in the Pacific Northwest. Up until that time, I'd been a backpacker and a mountaineer all my life. Obviously, when you go into the mountains with your things on your back, you pack your bag so that you've got the least weight possible. So I did the same thing for the kayak trip. I get to the west coast of Vancouver Island where we're about to start on this five-day trip, and I look out the corner of my eye at people unloading their cars. And they're taking out Dutch ovens and black forest cakes and *War and Peace* and whole salmon. I suddenly realized: of course, the kayak carries all the weight. In the buoyancy and fluidity of the water, you can carry 250 pounds in that kayak and you'll hardly notice it. I feel the same way about conversation now. You can allow a conversation to actually carry the weight of change.

When people go in to work, not only are they asked for more of their time, not only are they asked to be more responsible, to be more participative, but they're asked to change while they're at it. There's a part of us that says, 'Give me a break. With everything I have to do, I have to change at the same time?' In the middle of a talk at a telephone company in northern New York State a couple of years ago, I heard myself saying, 'No one has to change.' There was a moment of stunned incomprehension in the room, then this huge gale of laughter. The CEO had been in that morning saying, 'Everyone has to change.' What I meant was that no one has to change, but everyone has to have the conversation. Quite often in a workplace you will have enormous dynamics affecting the company. I've seen this again and again, from Fortune 500 companies down to the smallest kind of boutique advertising company. You will have

Tom Gegax

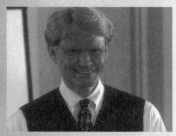

P R O F I L E

For entrepreneur Tom Gegax, the job description for "human being" includes two key functions: teaching and learning. It's a lesson he absorbed early in life from a favorite line of his dad's: "It's what you learn *after* you know it all that really counts."

In 1976, not yet 30 and with a family to support, Gegax took what he had learned from working for eight years at a major oil company, borrowed $60,000 and opened three tire outlets in Minneapolis. Twenty-two years later, Gegax is CEO of Team Tires Plus, the sixth largest independent tire store chain in the U.S., with sales in 1998 of $175 million.

His current success has been hard-won, with many ups and downs for both Gegax and the company. "In 1989, I had a three-ring wake-up call: divorce, a cancerous lump, and big financial problems for the company. It took that to make me ask, 'What's going on? I'm not leading others very well, and my relationships, while they appear good, evidently are not,'" Gegax remembers. "So I sought emotional and psychological growth through a therapist. I went there thinking I'll just go for a short time and find out what's wrong with everybody else; they must be causing the problem. Of course, I ended up learning a lot about myself."

That psychological journey prompted him to take a long hard look at what really mattered to him. "I came to believe that there's something I'm here to do, that I have a mission on the planet. The most important thing in my life is achieving that mission, my assignment from the universe. If I'm able to be a beneficial presence in the world in the ways I believe I'm assigned, then everybody wins. Just like if you achieve your personal mission, everybody wins."

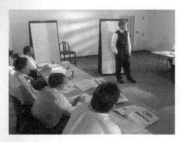

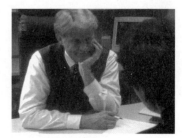

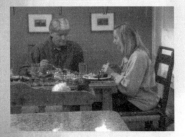 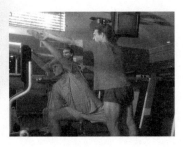 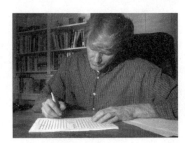

It's a personal philosophy that Gegax has incorporated more and more into his company's culture. "To have that mission be in alignment with your work mission makes it really fun. It's a good thing, obviously, when you don't have to wear one mask at home and another mask at work. The more congruent you can be, the less duality there is between workplace and home, the healthier that it is for everybody.

"But first, leaders need to do their own work. In other words, are they being real? Are they bringing that realness to both their personal and business lives? Secondly, are they creating an environment where others can do that? Or are they just saying they are, but the words are empty. You need to create an environment where people can challenge other people, where people are open to say what they feel, and there's a sense of freedom, even though certain kinds of structures need to be in place. Business should be done more consciously, in a more evolved manner, in a more enlightened manner."

For Gegax, an enlightened approach means treating employees as whole human beings, whose minds, bodies and spirits are connected. "I think most of the practices companies can implement to enhance the health of their employees—whether it's intellectual, physical, or psychological health—create an environment that's good for the health of the spirit. We're not talking about bringing religion into the workplace, by the way. That's a very important differentiation. We're talking about letting spirituality come forth, in an environment where people can be loving and caring, and have their spirit soar."

Over the years, Gegax has made certain lifestyle changes he felt enhanced his own health and energy levels, including practicing meditation and yoga, getting shiatsu massage, and gradually adopting a vegetarian diet. He found himself wanting to share the benefits with his staff. "It's very hard to feel spiritual if you're stressed, so we offer programs at our facilities that can help people manage their stress.

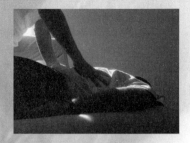

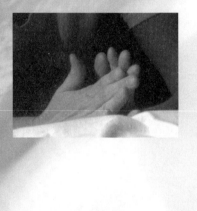

We bring speakers in to talk about psychology or spirituality. We have a workout room, and a meditation room for people who might want to do that. We offer shiatsu, nutritional cooking classes, smoking cessation.

"But I'm very aware that introducing complementary approaches into the company needs to be done gently. What I've tried to do is expose people to them, but never to push it. First of all, nobody would go for it. Second of all, it wouldn't feel right. I wouldn't have liked it, if it were me. So there are many, many different things. It's like a buffet. Do you like this? Do you not like that? Do you not like any of it? Great. No problem. We still love you.

"You don't offer these things to get great payback, you do them because it's right. Typically, companies will think of the costs instead of the benefits. Even within our company, there are times when we get challenged about the cost: 'Do we really need to do that for our people?' But I just think you can't lose. If you're helping your people, then they're going to be happier; therefore, there's going to be a lower turnover. They're going to be more productive and take fewer sick days. So there are all kinds of benefits for the company, but the biggest benefit is the smile on the face and the spring in the step."

Despite his business success and personal growth, Gegax is the first to admit that nobody's perfect. On the learning curve of life, he—and his company—are in there with the rest of us. These days he learns from his children, too. As his eldest son, Trent, tells him: "Dad, if you're not falling, you're not skiing."

dynamics affecting the company which no one dares speak about. They're hidden underneath. You'll have a three-hour meeting and the whole dynamic pushing the meeting will never be mentioned once. It's like the surface of a lake, below which no one will go.

HARRIS: You mentioned the need for the individual to have courage in the workplace. Is that also important to the company, to the employer? Is it valuable to them to have individuals who have the courage to speak up?

WHYTE: I think it is valuable today. You no longer have a world outside that is predictably heading in a certain direction like we had in the 1950s. You could think of the 1950s business world as a kind of monoculture, like a

Kansas wheat field. You've got one crop planted and that was the North American economy, the only one which survived the conflagration of the Second World War. There was an even keel to the world's competitive ambience at that time, which has totally disappeared. Now you have thousands and thousands of companies all the way around the world, all working in the same area that you are working in. Instead of a Kansas wheat field, we have a rain forest, and in a rain forest everything belongs exquisitely to the place where it lives. Every company now has to belong in an exquisite way to the place, to its function in the world, to its gift, to its service, to its product. It has to be very sharp and very alive. You can't get that aliveness and that adaptability unless you have individuals in your company who have their eyes and their ears open, who are looking out at the world and able to say, 'Hey, we can't do this anymore, because this is happening out in the world.' In a company where there's fear, you will not say we can't do this anymore, because saying that could threaten someone's identity—someone whose job description or title depends on your doing it the way it's always been done. It points up the need in business today for constant, courageous conversation.

HARRIS: So when individuals don't speak up, then the company ultimately fails.

WHYTE: It can. That's a magnified version of it. More often, the lack of courage leads to a slow demise.

HARRIS: You've written: 'The belief is that we can only enjoy life in the two-week intervals of vacation, and the rest of the time watch our souls shrivel as we spend our lives doing what we don't really want to do.' That sounds pretty awful. And yet thousands, maybe millions, of people would say they know exactly what you're talking about.

WHYTE: That's right. Obviously, there are many people who are very happy in their jobs. But I wanted to draw it in those bleak terms, because I think that almost everyone in their work life comes across a situation, at one time or another, where that negative dynamic is in place. Then they feel as if life is receding like a tide, and the vitality they had in their youth will never be available to them again. In effect, we're always going through a kind of mid-life crisis. A human being always has to reclaim their life by remembering what they're about, and poetry has a tremendous way of reminding us of that.

One of my poems is called "Loaves and Fishes." People find the first line very heretical. It shocks people, especially at high-tech companies.

This is not the age of information.
*This is **not***
the age of information.
Forget the news,
and the radio,
and the blurred screen.
This is the time
of loaves
and fishes.
People are hungry,
and one good word is bread
for a thousand.

The poet's question has always been: what is your one good word? What is the word in the next sentence, in the next conversation, that will break apart your identity and free you into a much larger territory in which you can be surprised, in which you can live again and not just endure.

HARRIS: On a practical level, how do we go about creating that kind of life for ourselves, the kind of work life that really does sustain us and nurture us and make us want to get up and be there in the morning.

WHYTE: First of all, you start a conversation inside yourself. You start a conversation about what you really want, and you dare to believe that it's all right to want what you want. You look at your desires as a kind of independent phenomena. You just allow them to be. You look at how they play out in your life, even though you won't give them voice on the surface. They're driving so much of what you do, so just engage in a conversation with them. You start to find that your own gifts are linked to your desires, so this is not a selfish exploration. You're exploring what you want, because you realize that there's no way you can have enthusiasm or any sense of what other people need in the world, unless you have some kind of link to your own wants in the world.

In my experience with many companies, it's amazing how you get the feeling that the only person that exists is the person in question, who sees all the other people who work there as simply highly paid extras in his or her career drama. That somehow God has arranged everything so that he or she can take the next step on the career ladder. It's a hugely mature thing for a human being to acknowledge that another person has a life of their own, and that they are also guided by their own stars. You can't grant that to another person unless you've granted that birthright memory to yourself. If you have given away your own desires in the workplace, it will be very hard for you to enthuse about someone else's plans or have a real conversation with anyone else.

People in the workplace have an immensely accurate and God-given B.S. detector. When it goes off, it's accurate down to parts of a billion. It goes off inside us when we hear someone, a boss, or whoever it is, in the workplace, asking us for qualities which they're not prepared to give themselves. They're asking for passion, and they have no passion themselves. They're asking for adaptability, and they're the least adaptable people around. And therefore, I will not join in their conversation. On the surface I will pay obeisance and say, 'Yes, of course,' but the part of me that's worth anything in the workplace is off somewhere else—usually in the bathroom talking with my colleagues about how unauthentic this all is.

But as soon as we realize that the person who's asking us for those qualities is attempting them themselves, then we're compelled. We don't need Shangri-la in the workplace. We're not looking for a 100 percent human-potentialized, California-hot-tub human being as our leader. What we need is someone who is attempting in their own life, no matter how humbly, to live out some of the qualities that they're asking from us. Then I'll join with them, if they ask me to, because I know that this is real. It's not simply a shell game that's being played.

HARRIS: It seems that as corporations try to do things differently, they take any number of approaches. They'll want to give out more vacation, or they'll want to have more office parties. They'll come in and paint the walls and put up more art or plants, things that are completely off the point of what you're talking about.

D
E
S
I
R
E
S

"If you have given away your own desires in the workplace, it will be very hard for you to enthuse about someone else's plans or have a real conversation with anyone else."

WHYTE: I'm not saying that organizations shouldn't reward their people. Give the vacations, give the prizes, paint the walls, provide the right environment, but most of all, be real with your people. I think one of the things that occurred when the Berlin Wall fell was that we suddenly realized that the nearest thing we had to an Eastern European dictatorship was a Western corporation. It was the place where we were told that this is not a democracy. It was the place where you had to toe the line. Now that world is falling away, just as the Berlin Wall fell away.

There's a kind of people-power now in the workplace that's equivalent to the people being out on the street in the Philippines, except it happens in much smaller doses in workplaces all around the country. We have a whole Generation X, and the generation that's now coming up behind them, that is impatient with that kind of structure. They have a totally different expectation of the world, and it doesn't have the same emphasis on predictability and structure as the '50s generation inherited coming out of the Depression and the Second World War.

HARRIS: Which is why you say that the 21st century will not be business as usual.

WHYTE: I think it's already not business as usual but certainly the changes will be going out in a much wider form, rippling out through all of our workers. I already feel, for instance, in the 12 years I've been in the work world, that there have been enormous changes. For instance, 11 or 12 years ago, there was still an argument around as to whether you should coerce your people into work or whether you should encourage them. That argument is over now. There's almost no one except for a few hard-headed dinosaurs who actually say that coercing people is a great thing, because we know that it's not sustainable. Eventually you pay for it; the people will make sure you pay for it. They'll refuse to bring the best part of themselves through the door.

REAL

"I'm not saying that organizations shouldn't reward their people. Give the vacations, give the prizes, paint the walls, provide the right environment, but most of all, be real with your people."

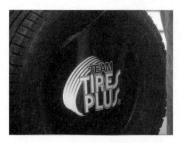
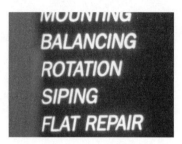
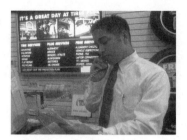

HARRIS: Why is it important for us to bring our best selves into the workplace?

WHYTE: It's important from a personal point of view, because we spend so much time in the workplace. It's important from the company's point of view, because in today's world you've got to be tremendously alert and adaptable to remain on the frontier of your own industry or business. You can't do it if your company and your people are asleep at the wheel. The company should be asking all the time, 'What is the conversation we're not having?' and individuals should be doing the same thing. If I leave the best part of myself in the car in the parking lot before I go in, I'm going to be spending 40—and if I'm in management circles, 50, 60, 70—hours a week split from myself.

That is not a passive process. It's a corrosive process. It's a process that causes you to distrust yourself and your world, and forget what's most precious to you. It has immensely poisonous effects on us. One of the things I've experienced in the workplace is that the people who are most cynical are actually the people who are the most idealistic, but they've had a terrible disappointment along the way at some time or another. They're the people who can stand up in a room and take all the energy out of it immediately, as you try to build anything. They said to themselves years ago, 'I cannot live out what is most precious to me in this workplace, so whenever I hear a conversation where people are actually acting as if you can do that, I'm going to stop it, because it makes me very angry. But underneath, it makes me very sad.' It's simply that they came, I think, to an erroneous conclusion that they could not do what was right in the workplace. They could not be themselves.

HARRIS: So what would you say to an individual who feels absolutely trapped in an oppressive work environment, when there's no place to go and bills to pay. What does that person do?

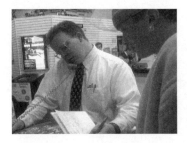 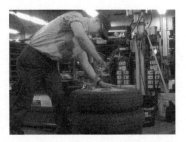 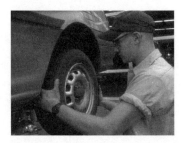

W H Y T E : Start talking to yourself. Start awakening parts of yourself. For a start, you're probably exhausted already. Start a conversation that actually starts to fire you up a little bit inside, you know. Then you start that conversation with someone else on the outside. Sometimes there's no one you can talk to in the workplace, no one you trust. Sometimes, even in your own family, there's no one you can talk to. So just start wherever you can. You open up with a stranger on a flight to Cincinnati, or at the Greyhound bus station, and you start to overhear yourself say things that you can't go back on. You start pushing yourself to articulate what you want, and once you've said it, it's out in the world. Then, little by little, you start to bring it into your workplace. You start doing little things, say, with friends, that are courageous, just saying something that's true that you'd be slightly afraid to say. You start to bring that slowly into your workplace. If there's absolutely no room for it there, then you're better off somewhere else. Hopefully, by this time, you've realized that if you can get to the place where you're giving the best of yourself, there will be a place where you belong. The world will actually come to meet you and embrace you.

One of the frightening things about the soul—and I use the word soul quite precisely in a poetic sense, meaning the part of us that's intense and serious about how it belongs in the world—one of the frightening things about opening up a conversation with yourself is, we intuitively know that the soul would much rather fail at its own life than succeed at someone else's. And that goes counter to an enormous tidal force, in North America especially, around our ideas of what success is and what it means.

H A R R I S : It sounds like this is a prescription for people who aren't in more workaday jobs. If your task in life is to cook the hamburgers, or get the coal out of the ground, or install the telephone, how do you instill that work with the kind of joy and courage that you're talking about?

WHYTE: There are many manual jobs that have far more skill than we normally associate with them. My own father, for instance, was an electrical cable jointer, as they're called in England. I worked with him many times and saw the amount of skill that is needed to do that kind of work. I also think that people who we normally associate with just wanting to get the work done, are actually crying out to be more involved. In many of the initiatives which have gone through the car industry in Detroit, I've brought people into quality circles or into discussions that previous generations of management said they were not fit for. Quite often, we're using very, very little of the people that we have working with us or for us. And the invitation itself opens up all kinds of wonderful surprises. If you don't make that invitation, you'll never find out what your people have to offer you. If you do make the invitation, and they're not willing to give it, you find out anyway what kind of people you have with you.

HARRIS: How would you define a soul-based workplace? Is there such a thing?

WHYTE: I think there is one, yes. It's a place where you're asking for people's gifts in the best way you can. A soul-based workplace asks things of me that I didn't even know I had. It's constantly telling me that I belong to something large in the world. I believe that human beings are desperate, always, to belong to something larger than themselves. When they don't feel that belonging, they not only feel as if they're running in place, they actually feel as if they're dying in place. A sure sign of a soul-based workplace is excitement, enthusiasm, real passion, not manufactured passion, but real involvement. And there's very little fear.

HARRIS: How do you answer the CEO who says, 'This is all well and good, and I'm sure it's even true, but my first responsibility is to my shareholders and my profits.' What do you say to him or her?

SOUL-BASED

---

*"A soul-based workplace asks things of me that I didn't
even know I had. It's constantly telling me that I belong to
something large in the world."*

WHYTE: I run into it increasingly less because in a sense the CEO stands at the crossroads between their people and their shareholders, too. But I'd say that having a participative workforce is great for business.

I believe that we are going through a difficult and wonderful place in the workplace right now, where all of our identities, our previously solid identities, are flowing away, and we're not yet sure who's there. We're not sure what the new workplace is, how we're supposed to be, and how our identities are actually configured. I wrote this poem called "The Journey" for a friend who was going through a difficult time. But it could also describe these threshold times we're facing in the new workplace. It's a poem that gives a flavor of how I work. I use it around change, because it has to do with pivoting our identity from the past to what's meeting us out there now. It's full of the imagery of the northwestern island near Seattle where I live.

Above the mountains
the Geese turn into
the light again

painting their
black silhouettes
on an open sky.

Sometimes everything
has to be
enscribed across
the heavens

so you can find
the one line
already written
inside you.

Sometimes it takes
a great sky
to find that

small, bright
and indescribable
wedge of freedom
in your own heart.

Sometimes with
the bones of the black
sticks left when the fire
has gone out

someone has written
something new
in the ashes of your life.

You are not leaving
you are arriving.

I think that it's incredibly useful right now for us to pivot ever so slightly from being held by our past notions of work, to pivot ourselves into the future by meeting that frontier, and not to look for ways to be kept in the manner to which we've become accustomed. More and more we're going to be asked to know what our gifts are, how we work best in the world. The next step is to come out from behind yourself, and start asking questions that put you at the frontier, not only of the way work is changing, but at the frontier of how you'll give your gift in the world through that work. I do think that we may be leaving this old workplace—but even more importantly, we're arriving at a new place.

TERAH COLLINS

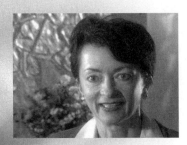

Terah Kathryn Collins is a nationally known consult-ant, speaker, and teacher of Feng Shui. She brings a background in communications and holistic health to her work with both residential and business clients. Collins is the author of *The Western Guide to Feng Shui: Creating Balance, Harmony, and Prosperity in Your Environment.*

BODY & SOUL: What is Feng Shui?

COLLINS: Feng Shui is a Chinese art and science that's over 3,000 years old. It's the study of how to arrange an environment to enhance the quality of someone's life. The words Feng Shui literally mean 'wind' and 'water.' It's a study of the seen, which is water, and the unseen, which is wind, and the relationship between the two. That relationship is what we address because what's going on inside of people's minds—their thoughts, emotions, and attitudes—is being stimulated by the seen, or what's in their environment.

BODY & SOUL: So the seen and the unseen is sort of a metaphor, where the unseen is what's happening internally in the person?

COLLINS: Right. It's about what's happening internally and how the envi-ronment is an externalization of that. When an environment is out of har-mony, it tends to drag a person's thoughts and associations and attitudes out of alignment or harmony, too. We want to lift the *chi*, or vital energy, in our homes and our workplaces by surrounding ourselves with things that lift us and have positive associations of all kinds.

BODY & SOUL: Tell me about the concept of *chi*.

COLLINS: *Chi* is a Chinese word that means vital energy. There are three ways to look at *chi*. One is that everything on our planet is alive with vital energy. Secondly, this vital energy is connecting all of us. When I first started to study Feng Shui, I thought that when I was in my car alone, I was alone, and if I was in my house alone, I was alone. The philosophy of *chi* says we are never alone, we are always connected to each other, and so relationship becomes very important. *Chi* is connecting every single thing in our lives. If I am in a career that I hate, it's going to affect my entire life. If I have a career that I love, that accentuates and empowers the rest of my life. So *chi* is alive in everything, *chi* connects everything, and thirdly, the *chi* in everything is always changing. We live in a dynamic universe which is in partnership with us.

BODY & SOUL: How does the concept of *chi* work in the practice of Feng Shui?

COLLINS: Many of us believe that we and our houseplants and our pets and our friends are filled with some kind of energy, but everything else is just inanimate stuff; it doesn't count. When we look through Feng Shui eyes, we see that everything is alive. Objects are not only molecularly alive, which we know through quantum physics, but they're also alive with our thoughts, feelings, associations. We have to address the *chi* in everything, in every piece of furniture, every article of clothing, every dish, because all of them are alive, and they're all talking to us in some way. Then the question becomes: are they saying nice things or not? We want to have things around us that have positive associations.

We can actually use our homes to anchor what it is we want, and where we want to go in life. Often, when people are trying to start a new business or they'd like a new relationship or they'd like to have a baby, their house is doing nothing to support them. It may be very extreme in its actual architecture, or uncomfortable, or very cluttered. That's where Feng Shui comes in, to create an environment that makes your heart sing. That is the essence of Feng Shui.

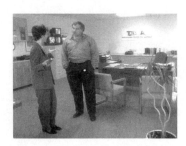
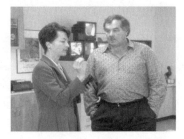
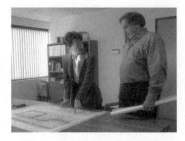

BODY & SOUL: It sounds like the principles of Feng Shui are basically about good architecture and good interior design, all good common sense that's been systematized based on these fundamental notions.

COLLINS: Feng Shui definitely reflects the true sense of common sense, which is based on survival, on figuring out how to place ourselves on the planet in a place that's the safest and most comfortable possible. It's also based on good interior design. All of the interior designers that have been through our Feng Shui school say that they learned a lot of this in their classes in interior design, or they've discovered a lot of these principles on their own. In fact, I find that there is a huge population of people who practice good Feng Shui intuitively. So, yes, common sense and good design principles are part of it. But what I find so intriguing is that it goes further than that to address the very nature of creation. We're looking at what the outer environment is saying about the inner being that's living there. Many times the outer environment will show exactly what the quality of that person's life is. So it goes deeper. It's the investigation of how can I bring in the inner development of the person. That's what people find very exciting.

BODY & SOUL: So when you go to a place to consult about Feng Shui, what do you do?

COLLINS: Usually people who call for a Feng Shui appointment have some kind of unhappiness, some place in their lives that's not working. I need to find out where the problem is in their lives. Then I look at their environment to see where I can find what I call the environmental splinter—or what is matching and holding in place this unhappiness. Feng Shui is the belief that the external reality affects the internal reality. So I look for how the unhappiness is expressed environmentally and change it for the better. Then I watch to see

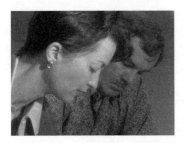
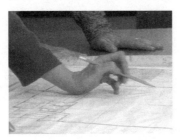
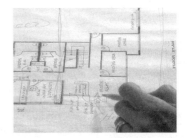

what happens in their lives, because if it makes no difference, why in the world would we be practicing Feng Shui? We're practicing it because it is effective. When we do change that external problem or challenge, what will almost always happen is a great improvement in the quality of these people's lives.

BODY & SOUL: We've been talking mostly about personal spaces. When you work with corporations and companies, what are business people looking for from Feng Shui?

COLLINS: When I'm working with a corporation, the same principles are put into action. We're creating an environment where the employees and the customers maintain a sense of comfort and safety. When a person is well-versed in Feng Shui, they become excellent at seeing all of the details that are being registered on a subconscious level by most people. All of us are making judgments all of the time. For instance, I worked with a craft gallery where the displays were set up so that the corners of the pedestals all faced toward the door. This will actually tend to push customers away. They'll stand at the door and say, 'Well, I'm not sure I want to go in there,' and keep on walking. But if we turn the pedestal cases so that there's a flat surface facing the door, that signals a welcome to customers. These are environmental cues that are saying 'yes' rather than saying 'no.'

Similarly, in a corporation, you can put all yes's into the architecture and the design, rather than either a mix of yes and no, or all no's. I've worked with many places that were trying to do business—and the office is full of dead plants. Or there are all kinds of problems with the way people are facing or the way their work stations are put together. These are not optimum conditions, yet everyone is expected to do excellent work and get great results. And that just doesn't happen. Human beings don't respond well to terrible environments. Feng Shui practitioners know how to correct environments that are that way,

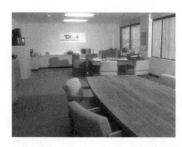
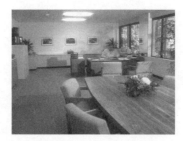
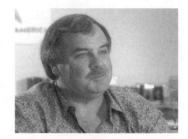

many times without having to spend a lot of money. Oftentimes, it's more about placement than about replacement.

BODY & SOUL: So it sounds like if you understand your client well and their relationship to their physical environment, you'll give them a sense of peace and comfort. That doesn't sound like the sort of mystical witchcraft that a lot of Western people who don't understand what Feng Shui is, may take it to be.

COLLINS: Feng Shui has so much of value to give us in our Western culture. There's a lot of Feng Shui that's practiced following the Eastern traditions, and they're quite beautiful. However, there's a whole population of people who would like to experience Feng Shui without having to get involved with all of the Eastern traditions, and they don't have to. I absolutely believe in building rapport with every single person that I work with. The last thing I want to do is to turn someone off to the possibility of making a more wonderful environment for themselves. So it does not need to sound foreign or include a lot of foreign objects. We can use very familiar things to reorient and establish *chi* flow, so that no matter who comes in, no one would know it's been 'Feng Shui-ed.' All they know is that they feel extremely comfortable in that environment and happy to do business with that company.

BODY & SOUL: Can you explain the connection between applying Feng Shui principles and a business making more money?

COLLINS: When a company wants to make more money, and we're looking at it through Feng Shui eyes, I will look at the flow of *chi* throughout the entire business. For example, there can be pockets throughout a business where it's full of clutter or it's completely discombobulated. I've done work with a company where they had 25 dead computers stashed away. They thought it didn't matter because they were hidden away in a back room, but in Feng Shui, every square inch counts. There's no such thing as a place to hide stuff. When we think there's a place to hide stuff, that stuff is usually in chaos. I go through with my Feng Shui eyes wide open and look for those places where the *chi* flow has stagnated or been stopped for some reason.

Businesses that are alive and successful, when you walk in, they're identified everywhere. They don't want you to forget who they are and why they're on the planet. So we want to do that with businesses. We want them to put their stake into the ground and claim their space and be ready to capture the success that they want. We want to remove discomfort and produce an environment that is very comfortable; and that also, on an instinctual level, feels safe and that people are happy to do business with. If it feels good to be there, business will happen.

BODY & SOUL: How do employees of a company come into this?

COLLINS: In Feng Shui, it's vital to honor every single human being that surrounds us. So when we are an owner of a business, every one of our employees needs to be honored. We honor them by placing them so that they can see what's going on, where they have natural elements and good lighting. We're meeting their basic requirements for a positive reason that makes sense to everybody. Because the happier an employee is, the less often they'll be sick, the more productive they'll be, and the more identified with their company they will be.

It's simple to do. People do not have huge requirements. When I go into a sea of cubicles, for instance, a lot of times there's no way we're able to reconfigure those work stations, but we can give everybody a small mirror, so that everyone can see behind them. That calms everyone down and it's so simple. A lot of Feng Shui sounds very simple, and yet the change can be profound. It's the tiny difference between a comfortable chair and an uncomfortable chair. That's actually a profound difference when you want an employee to be giving you their all.

BODY & SOUL: What do you see as the benefits of Feng Shui?

COLLINS: Feng Shui will benefit just about any facet of life—wealth and prosperity, our relationships in the community, our marriage, our relationship with our children or our friends, our career, our creativity, our health. Each one of those has an inner component that Feng Shui will begin to stimulate,

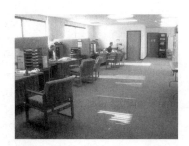
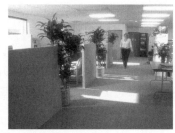
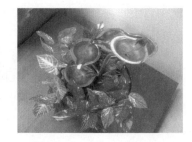

because we're always looking at that inner and outer relationship. For example, prosperity is so much more, so much bigger than cash in the bank. Riches have to do with being grateful for everything in our lives, anything from having our whole body to having our family, all of the things that money can't buy. So there are deeper lessons and deeper ways of thinking about each one of these treasures that Feng Shui will come in and give you. The outer work certainly starts the ball rolling, but the inner work is equally important.

A lot of times in this culture, we'll try to resist change, put the brakes on—only buy a sofa once in our lives, or pick one career and stick with it for our whole lives. Meanwhile, our lives are going by with tremendous and constant change. So, in Feng Shui, we're always suggesting to people that they embrace change and make friends with it, because change can always move us forward into a better and better place. We want to allow change to really operate for us, because that's bringing in the new *chi* and letting go of the old *chi*. I find that many times what I'm teaching people is how to exhale and let go and trust and allow, rather than always inhaling, taking in, consuming, and not letting go as fast as they might otherwise.

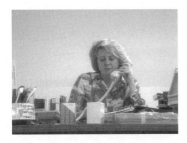 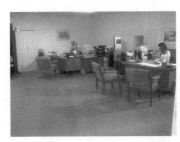 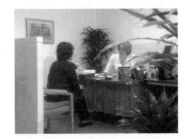

8 ODE TO JOY: WHY YOUR ATTITUDE MATTERS

There have been so many joys for me, personally, as I set about creating and then implementing the *Body & Soul* television series: Working with an incredibly talented group of producers and editors. Having lengthy conversations with (I believe) some of the most interesting doers and thinkers on the planet today. Sharing my excitement about these ideas with an ever-widening group of friends. Watching as colleagues at PBS stations across the country responded enthusiastically to the programs. As I keep telling my family, this project has yet to feel like work; it has all been a joy.

In many ways, this chapter summarizes my own outlook on life. I've always been an incorrigible optimist, so much so that not only is the glass always half-full, I'm convinced that there's someone around the very next corner with a brimming pitcher, just waiting to fill it up again.

Research tells us now that a joyous and optimistic attitude is not only good for our mental health, it's also good for our physical health. But if joy is so important, how can we achieve it? How do we go about keeping our spirits up amid a daily dose of news about events that seem frightening, horrifying, or both? How can we make sure we inject pleasure in our lives when we don't know how long the job will last, when the bills are mounting up, the baby's sick, or aging parents need more time than we can give them?

As you'll discover, it can be done. Sister Alice Williams finds strength, upliftment, and inspiration from the gospel music she shares with anyone willing to listen. Psychologist Stella Resnick suggests that happiness can begin with something as simple and accessible as taking a few deep, relaxing breaths. And author Sarah Ban Breathnach "excavates" for joy in the small moments of life, which she records faithfully in a gratitude journal.

Like many things that are worthwhile, however, consciously adding happiness to our lives doesn't come without effort. Sometimes a sunset is so breathtakingly glorious, we can't help but notice; other times, the sinking sun spreads the merest blush of pink across a darkening sky. Either way, appreciating the wonder of the daily celestial light show begins with remembering to open our eyes. If joy is the end result of appreciation, appreciation comes from paying attention.

The best news is that whoever we are, wherever we live, whatever the state of our bank account, making the effort to connect with something larger than ourselves isn't so hard. You can start by going outside, taking a few deep breaths and looking up. It can be pretty dazzling, that sky. And it's there for us, all the time.

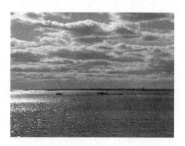

STELLA RESNICK

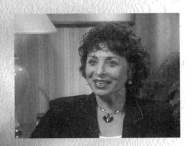

Stella Resnick, Ph.D., is a psychologist in private practice in Los Angeles, a frequent speaker at professional conferences, and the author of *The Pleasure Zone: Why We Resist Good Feelings & How to Let Go and Be Happy.*

HARRIS: I want to ask about this notion of the pursuit of happiness. Now, presumably that's important to us as Americans, since, after all, it's written in our Constitution. What is it, do you think, that makes so many people feel as if they shouldn't be pursuing it, that maybe they don't deserve to be happy?

RESNICK: Our culture really does not respect pleasure. Our culture thinks pain builds character and gives meaning to life, and that people who do pursue pleasure are selfish and self-centered and only out for their own good. In fact, nothing can be further from the truth. We really need to pursue fulfillment; we really need to be nourished in our lives. What happens is that as we're growing up, we are trained to hold ourselves back from feeling as good as we can because we're told to sacrifice, that to show our love for other people we really need to sacrifice ourselves, and we need to put other people first. The problem is that if we put other people first all the time, we lose the ability to enjoy our own lives, and then we're running on empty. We're depleted, we're doing things for other people, and we feel guilty when we're having too good a time.

HARRIS: How did you personally come to this notion that, in fact, it is not only okay to be happy, but it is important?

RESNICK: I had been in the best therapy with the best therapists for several years and I was not happy. I knew a lot about why I was unhappy; I knew a lot about my past background and how that had held me back. I knew about my anxiety, I knew about my shame, I knew about my guilt. I knew about injuries, I knew about my wounds. I knew all about it, but I was unhappy. So I took off a year from my life and I put myself into exile. I got myself a cabin in the woods in Woodstock, New York, and I started to really look at why I was so miserable. Despite all that I knew, and all the therapy that I'd been in, and the fact that I was a good therapist and doing good for others, still, I wasn't happy.

What I started to discover was that I wasn't happy because I didn't know how to be happy. I did not know how to take pleasure in my everyday life. I knew how to be entertained, I knew how to go to shows, I knew how to be 'on,' I knew how to go to parties. I knew how to succeed. I knew how to prove myself, and thought that that would give me happiness. Finally, I knew, at that point in my life, how to achieve material success. And still I wasn't happy.

When I put myself into retreat, I started to see that I was on my case all the time, that I was always critical about myself, that I was always regretting the past and anticipating a negative future. That's when I started seeing the importance of taking pleasure in everyday life, and how incapable I was of doing that.

Then when I started to research pleasure—because therapists know a lot about pain, but we know very little about pleasure—when I started to research this, I saw that nobody in psychology knew anything about pleasure, including Freud. Freud said that pleasure was nothing more than the absence of pain. Well, how do you define something by what it's not? I'm not a banana split, but that doesn't tell you what I am.

I'm thrilled that I have become an expert on pleasure, because what better thing can I leave as my legacy on the planet than a recognition of the importance of pleasure and, also, how to have it on a practical level. How to recognize that you're resisting it, how to recognize that we're trained to believe that even though the pursuit of pleasure is in our Constitution, we really don't feel entitled to it. And how important it is for our health.

HARRIS: One of the first steps, you say, is to let go of time. Why is that important?

RESNICK: Time regiments us. We do things by the clock. We wake up when we're supposed to, we have breakfast when we're supposed to, we get out of the house when we're supposed to. We meet our obligations that way and it's a way of pacing us to the larger culture, with the rhythm of the larger culture, and to our responsibilities. It makes us lose touch with ourselves. When I started to want to be in tune with myself, I had to turn the clocks around.

Otherwise, I was constantly focused on what I should do, when. When I turned the clocks around, when I taped over the clock on the stove, what I began to see was what I wanted to do, what were my natural rhythms. When did I want to have lunch—not that it was time for lunch, but when did I feel hungry—what I wanted to do next, and how long I wanted to read, and when I wanted to stop.

I started to tune in to my own desires, to my own urges. Being able to divorce yourself from the tyranny of time is such an important aspect. When we want to rest and relax and replenish ourselves, we have to let go of time, even if sometimes we give ourselves 20 minutes only. But those 20 minutes have to be free from time. Set a clock, or a timer, so that you know when the 20 minutes are up. There are times when I have half an hour to get somewhere, but I need to have a 10-minute bath. I can get into a bath and even though it's only 10 minutes long, I can forget about time for nine minutes and that's important.

HARRIS: There's another element of time, I think, which is that many people think that at some future point in their lives they will be happy: 'When I find the perfect mate, when I land the perfect job, when I finish school, when I get a great car,' whatever. Your point seems to be, don't wait for that, figure out ways to be happy now.

RESNICK: It's so important that we live our lives on a daily basis. Because, as I tell people, which in some ways is a comforting thought, you may not live long enough for your worst fears to come true. We do a lot of worst-case scenarios; we rehearse what we don't want to happen. It's very important for us to recognize that life is what's happening while we're busy making other plans, as John Lennon said. It is important for us to find pleasure in daily life.

R E P L E N I S H

"When we want to rest and relax and replenish ourselves, we have to let go of time."

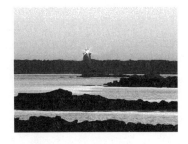

What frequently happens to people when they set goals for themselves is that they decide they will be happy when they achieve a particular thing. In order to get there, they do all kinds of bad things to themselves and put themselves through all kinds of turmoil. Then they discover that they have to keep that turmoil up in order to maintain whatever success they achieved in that tumultuous way. And so there's no escape from, 'At some future time, I will be happy,' because the habits that you have to get there are going to be habits that you're going to continually repeat. People who win the lottery and solve their financial problems, six months later are back to whatever misery they were in before they won the lottery and then some, because now they have troubles they didn't even know about.

So it's really important to do what you love to do, enjoy your days, dream of what it is that you want, work hard for it, but make sure that the work you're doing is work you love, that you enjoy what you're doing. That way, you may or may not achieve it; if you do, it's gravy. It's wonderful. But if you enjoy the process, then no matter what happens, whether you receive the rewards that you were hoping for or not, it won't have been a waste, because you really enjoyed the process of getting there.

HARRIS: It sounds so simple to say, basically, 'Relax and enjoy and let life happen'. That also means that you have to shut off that little voice in your head that's saying, 'Not enough. Not enough time,' or, 'I'm not doing this right.' All that sort of self-critical stuff that most of us feel whirling around in our heads all the time. How do you shut off that voice?

RESNICK: The key to everything, the secret to success in all things, is being able to relax during stressful or challenging times, and the key to that is the breath. We really need to be able to take deep inhales, and take long exhales, periodically through the day, so that we can relax ourselves. When we start to

BREATH

"The key to everything, the secret to success in all things, is being able to relax during stressful or challenging times, and the key to that is the breath."

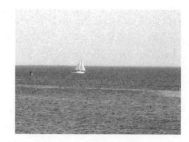

Mary Alice Williams

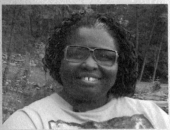

P R O F I L E

Some people seem to be born knowing how to make a joyful noise. For the rest of us, a little encouragement may be required.

Mary Alice Williams, known to her students as "Sister Alice," has been steeped in the gospel tradition of love, grace, and redemption since her childhood in Philadelphia. "Our house was always blasting with gospel music," she recalls. "I've always sung at the church, the choir, and in groups. It's just a part of my life."

For the past six years at the Omega Institute in upstate New York, she has been helping others discover the music within them—even if they've never encountered gospel before and certainly never imagined they could sing it for themselves. "As a little girl in church, music always made me feel happy, and music always made me think. Gospel music to me is about hope. Sometimes when I felt like there was no hope in some situations, it gave me the strength to pull myself together and move on out into bigger and better things.

"It's a gift God gave to my people because of the hard times that they've had to come through. I believe that's why our people are so strong. I believe the same hope it brought to them then, it brings to everybody now, not just to the African-Americans.

"Sometimes the tears will just flow and flow in class, because the message is getting in their heart and they're receiving the message. A lot of times after class, people come and talk to me and just tell me the appreciation they have for this music, and what it meant to them in this time in their life. There's not a week that goes past that I don't get a call from at least three to four people.

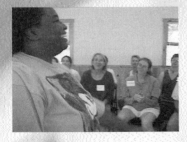
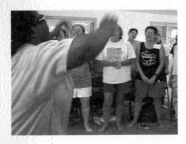
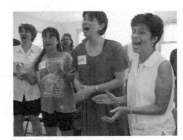

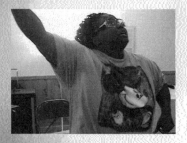 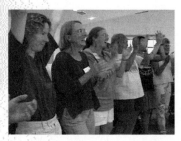 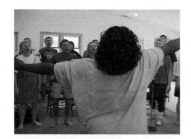

"Every time I stand up there and I see these people, it gives me energy, because I know they want to learn this gospel music, which has spread hope throughout generations and nationalities and cities and countries.

"This music does bring about a joy that makes your physical body respond to what you feel. It brings about a peace. It brings about a different focus on life. Gospel music is healing. It's healing to body, soul, and spirit."

relax ourselves, we start to really hear that critical inner voice. It's important that we recognize that critical inner voice is not a help to us.

That critical inner voice maintains us in stress, and it drives us through fear. Anything that drives us through fear is going to drive us to contraction, getting tight and small, and holding the breath, and being driven. When we operate in that way, we're not all that we can be, because all that we can be comes from being expansive, comes from being open, comes from being drawn to what excites us, rather than being driven by fear or driven by negativity. So it's really important that we recognize this inner voice, that we know that this inner voice comes, generally speaking, from a critical parent. Or, if we didn't have a critical parent, we make one up. We really don't need that.

One of the ways that I work with people with their critical inner voice—because I had one most of my life, and it held me back—what I recommend is to build another voice, what I call the voice of the inner ally. This is the voice of the kind, compassionate parent. This is the voice that says, 'You are good, you are smart, you can do it.' It's the voice of inner encouragement, the voice that reminds us to take deep breaths and relax, so that we can grapple with these difficulties. Because the critic does not help. But you can't get rid of something by stopping it, you can't force yourself to stop something. What you can do is notice it and be observant of how you're talking to yourself. Recognize that it's not going to do you any good. Invoke a higher voice, and learn how to use that voice to inspire and encourage yourself.

HARRIS: Is there a connection in your mind between happiness and health?

RESNICK: Oh, there's a very big connection. We have lots of data to show that people who are fulfilled in their lives, who have more good experiences, closeness with family and good friends and pets, and feel fulfilled in their work—the essential elements of happiness—these are the people who tend to resist illness, even illness that they're genetically predisposed toward. We have plenty of evidence to show that.

These are also people who, when they do get ill, recover faster. There's a lot of good evidence to show that the happier we are, the healthier we are. And often, too, the healthier we are, the happier we'll be, too.

HARRIS: You've actually written that happiness prolongs life. Really?

RESNICK: Yes, we see so many people who are creative in their lives, living very long, fulfilling lives. Beatrice Wood, a ceramist, who recently died at the age of about 104, every day was an adventure to her. Up until her last days, she woke up every morning and dressed in her beautiful Indian saris and made herself up and wore all her jewelry. Life was exciting to her; she wanted to live. People who are creative, people who are connected, tend to live longer than people who aren't.

I had a great-aunt who used to travel from Brooklyn to Manhattan twice a week to do volunteer work with the aged. When she told me about that, she

F U L F I L L M E N T

"People who are fulfilled in their lives, who have more good experiences, closeness with family and good friends and pets...these are the people who tend to resist illness."

herself was 89 years old, and she was travelling by subway to do volunteer work with 'the old people'. I said to her, 'Aunt Henya, what are you, if not old?' She said, 'Well, I'm more fortunate than the others.' But I believe that her good fortune was her big heart and her desire to do good. She loved her life. And when you love life, you tend to live longer.

HARRIS: You also mention touch, play, laughter, movement. How do they create happiness?

RESNICK: Well, they create happiness because they enable us to be nourished and fulfilled. Touch is a very important element of fulfillment, in the sense that it connects us with other people. When we're in pain, the most healing thing that somebody can do for us is touch us. Give us a hug, give us a touch, give us a squeeze, and we know that. We automatically do that with someone. If someone is telling us about something that causes them pain, we automatically reach out and touch or embrace them.

All the different ways you've mentioned stimulate our nervous system in such a way that enables us to open up. We have a nervous system that is in two parts: the sympathetic and parasympathetic system. The sympathetic governs fight-or-flight; the parasympathetic side is love and pleasure; and they kind of work antagonistically. When we're in pain, everything contracts and closes down. We hold the breath and adrenaline shoots through the body. When we're feeling pleasure, we take a deep breath, we open up and everything relaxes. There's energy flow and that happens on a physical level, on a body level. The muscles relax, the blood vessels open. If blood is rushing through the blood vessels—rather than when we're in pain, and the blood vessels are really tight and the pressure builds—obviously there are going to be more nutrients being brought to our tissues and organs and more waste products being removed, because everything is flowing more easily. So there is a very keen connection between touch and laughter and meditation and exercise, particularly if you enjoy it. Singing and kissing and making love—all of that stimulates the parasympathetic nervous system, which opens everything up and allows energy flow, which is really the basis of healing.

HARRIS: Is this something that should come naturally?

RESNICK: It doesn't come naturally to us because of our social conditioning from people who think that we have to work hard to suppress everything, who think we're born evil. The people who think we're born good, believe that

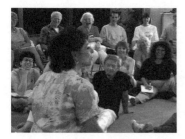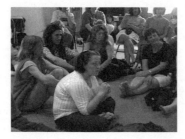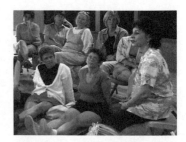

all we need to do is be nourished and relaxed, and that we will be able to do good. But we're out of touch with how to do that. What we really need to learn is how to channel our energies. We don't have to repress ourselves to be good. Nor can we just say, 'Well, the hell with everything, the hell with you, I'm just going to pursue my own pleasure,' because then you're going to be all alone. Nobody's going to want to hang out with you because you're so selfish and self-centered. So the important thing to recognize is that we need to share our pleasures. We need to learn how to do that. It takes a certain amount of discipline. You cannot just do it by becoming determined to have as good a time as you can and everything else be damned. It doesn't work that way.

HARRIS: You've written: 'How you choose to talk to yourself will determine your mood and affect your health and immunity.' That sounds a little startling. How you talk to yourself affects your immunity?

RESNICK: Yes, definitely. If you talk to yourself in harsh tones, you're going to stimulate the sympathetic nervous system, and that's going to tighten your heart and create all kinds of fears and anxieties. Because how do we talk to ourselves when we're negative? We're saying, 'You're never going to get anywhere, no matter what you do. You're going to be alone, you're never going to find somebody to love you. You're not good enough for the work that you're doing, you have to work harder.' So what happens when we do that? We stimulate the sympathetic nervous system; we're in fight-or-flight; we are living on adrenaline; we become adrenaline junkies. Then we have to jack ourselves up, because what happens with adrenaline is that it jacks you up but then it drops you and you feel spent. So now you've got to use drugs or alcohol to get yourself back up there. That is all going to affect your immunity.

What you want to be able to do is stimulate yourself to be excited in your life. To be enthusiastic. To be curious, to care about things. To be motivated out of

Sarah Ban Breathnach

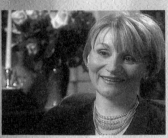

P R O F I L E

Sarah Ban Breathnach (pronounced Bon Brannock) lives in a quiet neighborhood just outside Washington, D.C. There is nothing about the townhouse to proclaim that a mega-best-selling author makes her home here. But anyone who has read and appreciated the ideas she writes about in *Something More: Excavating Your Authentic Self* and *Simple Abundance:A Daybook of Comfort and Joy* would instantly recognize these surroundings as hers.

The living room furniture is upholstered in chocolate brown velvet, with "Embrace Life" stenciled in gold paint over the fireplace. The words "Serenity," "Wisdom," and "Harmony" appear elsewhere around the house. Carefully arranged fresh flowers brighten a chest in the entrance hall and add color to a lushly draped table in the living room. All around the room are framed family pictures, and a variety of objects from the thrift shops she loves to frequent.

It is a warm and intensely personal space, assembled over time with the kind of care and attention Ban Breathnach urges the rest of us to bring to the details of our lives. But she is more than the "Martha Stewart of the spiritual set," as she has been described. Her attentiveness to life's little moments came at a considerable cost, more than a dozen years ago. Then a freelance writer and radio journalist, Ban Breathnach was sitting at a fast-food restaurant with her two-year-old daughter Katie, when suddenly a large ceiling panel dropped onto her head.

"Thank God that I took the blow and Katie didn't, because they say it would have killed her. But I had a concussion, and I was partially disabled for 18 months after that. It was one of the darkest times in my life. I actually think of it now as a death. It was a death of the life that I had planned. I had to learn life all over again. I couldn't read. I couldn't listen to music because I couldn't make sense of it. I couldn't have telephone calls. Even the pattern on the quilt made me dizzy; we had to turn the quilt over so I could just look at the plain muslin backing. And also we tried to keep it a secret, because if you're a freelance writer and radio broadcaster, nobody wants to hire somebody who has had a head injury."

Out of this life-transforming event came a new attitude and, eventually, a new career. As she slowly began to recover, Sarah recalled, "I became grateful for every little thing: if I had been able to listen to a snatch of music and not get sick or dizzy. To be able to go downstairs and not be wobbly, and make a cup of tea. To go out into the back yard and see the falling leaves, or even in December to see the slant of light that Emily Dickinson talks about, things that were so minute that I had never taken time to notice before."

She began to document all those moments in a "gratitude journal." "I would write them down because I would forget them. And it wasn't just short-term memory loss from the head injury. I would write them because I would forget them from the frenzy of life. I mean, so many things can happen to you that are very pleasant during two hours, but by the end of the day you don't remember.

"One of the wonderful things is to go back and look at your gratitude journal after several months, or even a year, and see that it's not the big moments that are the things that really count, it's the small moments. We think that it's the promotion, the new baby, the new house, the big moments in life; we think that's what life is. But when you look back at a gratitude journal, you've given thanks for the way the dining room looks because you've washed the windows and the sunlight is coming in now. Or after you have that baby, just sitting and playing with him, and so you write that down: 'We had a wonderful 15 minutes playing, or building blocks.'

"Then you see that it's the small things that are the sacred moments, and they form the narrative of our lives. That is when joy comes into your life, because joy is a spiritual gift that doesn't depend on external events."

Despite her recent financial success, she still relies on the simple things of life to bring her pleasure: flower arranging, tending to her patio garden, looking for hidden treasures inside thrift and antique shops, writing in her journal. "If you wake up in the morning and you say, 'I'm going to have five things when I go to bed tonight to be

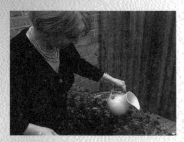
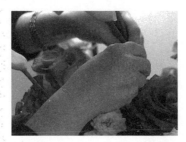
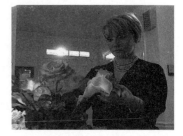

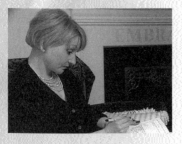
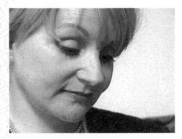
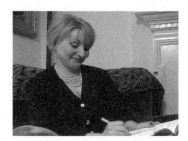

grateful for, that made my life interesting today,' you won't go to bed the same person."

Another one of her spiritual experiments has been tithing—the Biblical tradition of giving back a tenth of what is received. Even before she became a best-selling author, she decided to test the concept to see what would happen. "I started to tithe my grocery money. I started to tithe whatever little check came in. And when you don't have money, you think that when you get a check for a hundred dollars, 'Oh, my God, I can't give 10 dollars away because I've got all these bills to pay.' That is exactly the time you should start tithing.

"Ever the skeptic, I would make a note of how things would go, and I discovered something interesting. When I gave away a tenth—it could be to a church, or to an organization that was doing good work—I noticed that the money that I did have, lasted longer. And when I didn't tithe, the boiler would break down, the car would need a new muffler—I mean, something would happen and it would be more money than the tithe money. So I noticed this pattern, and I thought, 'Hmm, this is very fascinating.' But by that time I had started to give, and I liked the feeling, so I continued."

Sarah also tries to remain connected to nature as a way to keep joy in her life. "I open my eyes, and I look, and I discover a spider spinning a web. And instead of just smacking it down, I let it spin the web. I listen to the birds sing, and I hear that there are five different concertos going on outside the bedroom window. And I believe in sacred idleness, too, just sitting down underneath a tree, and taking a deep breath and 'being.' I love the fact that we are called, not 'human doings,' but 'human *be*-ings.' That is the one thing that most of us have great difficulty with, just being. If we could just 'be' who we are, to ourselves and to each other, we would know joy all the time."

positive energy, rather than negative energy. That positive energy stimulates the parasympathetic system, opens everything up. It stimulates endorphins, and we know that there is a connection between endorphins and other neuropeptides in the system, and health. All of that helps us to repair our systems, which is what healing is about. Healing is about repair, replenishment, rebirth, renewal. In order to be able to do that, we need to be open, we need to have energy, we need to be enthusiastic about life. To repair means to be at one with yourself, to mend wounds. To replenish means to bring in fuel and energy. And to be reborn means to let go of toxic parts of yourself that are not helping you to heal, and to let those parts slough off, so that you can renew yourself. All of that takes expansiveness, takes breathing, takes being relaxed and energized at the same time. That's my definition of vitality. If you think about it, when you feel the most vital, the most alive, you are energized, but you're relaxed at the same time. You can do anything, you can go anywhere, because you've got all this 'get up and go,' as they say.

HARRIS: There are those who say you can begin to find happiness by maintaining an 'attitude of gratitude,' being grateful for all the small moments in your day. Do you agree?

RESNICK: I definitely do. I think gratitude is a very healing emotion, because what happens when we're in stress is that we're thinking of all that we don't have. When our relationships aren't working, it's because we're focused on what we don't have with our partners, and it's very important to start to focus on what we do have. Gratitude is a wonderful way to focus on the great gift of life, and the great gift of what the people that we love give to us. Even though you may have had a difficult childhood, it's still very important to recognize that sometimes, even the people who unconsciously were abusive towards you still gave you some gifts.

ENTHUSIASM

"Healing is about repair, replenishment, rebirth, renewal. In order to be able to do that, we need to be open, we need to have energy, we need to be enthusiastic about life."

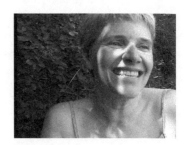

G R A T I T U D E

When you start to focus on being grateful, particularly when it's augmented by breath, then your heart will begin to open. When you start to feel grateful, when you're reminded of the people who have really benefited you in their life, you have their picture in your mind's eye and you can feel connected to them. In that moment, you are giving yourself a spurt of wonderful life force. So the more we can be grateful, the more we remember to be grateful, the more we thank God for what we have—the more we'll have.

HARRIS: I'm wondering if being a more joyful person also tends to make someone a more spiritual person.

RESNICK: I think so, because if you're more fulfilled in yourself, you tend to give more to others, because you have more to give. There's a tendency to want to share, there's a tendency to be compassionate, there's a tendency to be empathetic when you have suffered. When you know what kind of pain you've been through and how it feels, you're better able to identify with other people. To see someone in pain, if you've got more than they have, it makes you want to share. And all of these are very spiritual values.

I define spirituality as feeling a part of something good that's larger than yourself. That's what we feel when we are more joyful. We feel that we belong. You can't be joyful if you feel at odds with the culture at large. If you feel that there's nobody around that you can communicate with, you're not going to have joy. So being a joyful person, being a happy person, automatically says that you have good relationships. If you have good relationships, then you're going to extend yourself to people, even people you don't know, because you'll feel with them and that's what we mean by compassion.

HARRIS: Do you think that we as a culture or as a society are ready to hear this? Does this speak to something, perhaps, on some level that we already know, even if we haven't consciously thought about it?

"Gratitude is a very healing emotion, because what happens when we're in stress is that we're thinking of all the things we don't have. It's very important to start to focus on what we do have."

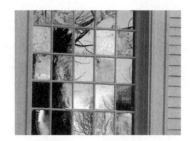

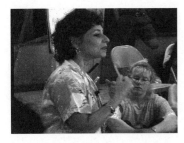 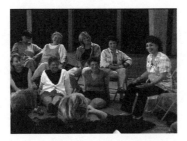

RESNICK: I think our culture is very ready for this. I think the fact that there's such a burgeoning interest in spirituality nowadays speaks to the need to feel a part of a community, because spirituality really is about community. It's about being connected. We need this right now. There's too much self-interest, there's too much stress and pain and infighting. There are all kinds of things that are going on in the world now, and a lot of people are getting sick of it. We're recognizing that it's such a pleasure, it feels so good, to be a part of a community of like-minded people, of people who want to do good for others, who want to share—people who want to have, for example, a quiet mind, and to be at peace within, where stress is no longer a way of life. People are beginning to recognize that even when they get the material goods that they want, it's not worth it if they have to be in stress to keep it.

It feels good to pray and be in contact with a higher source. Even if you don't believe in God, you can find that higher source within yourself that we're all connected to. It feels wonderful to do good for others, and to see the benefits of what you're doing. It is so inspiring and feels so good to come to terms with our mortality, and to fashion an afterlife that we can live by that gives us existential courage. These are all spiritual values. It's very important for us, now, to be able to deal with some of these things on a higher level.

HARRIS: Does it take a long time for someone to go from a place of unhappiness to a place of happiness?

RESNICK: It takes forever. By that, I mean that it doesn't take forever to feel happy, but it is a daily discipline. It's about waking up and counting your blessings instead of your curses, and looking at what it is that you have to be grateful for. Remind yourself when you're in a stressful place to breathe and relax, because that way you'll be able to grapple with the challenge of the moment and be able to recognize it. Even when you are in conflict with someone else, know that they're really not a bad person. Remind yourself to breathe and to relax, and to communicate in a gentle, loving way, rather than in an angry, forceful, violent way.

All of these skills take reminding ourselves constantly throughout the day, relaxing and breathing; taking time out for ourselves, quiet time; taking a moment to close your eyes and to meditate just for a minute, or to say a little prayer that will give you courage to move on. Those are the kinds of things that we really need to do on a daily basis. Being able to be fulfilled, being able to be happy is a lifestyle. It's not just an attitude change, because we forget.

I forget, you know. I wrote a book on pleasure, and yet I have to remind myself daily to breathe and to relax. I have to remind myself when something disappointing happens, or when I lose an opportunity, that another opportunity will come. I have to invoke my own inner ally. I have to give myself courage sometimes to face something that's difficult. I have to also remind myself to express my disappointment or my pain to somebody in a kind and generous way, rather than to be angry or vindictive. We have to do that daily. So how long does it take? All of our lives. But what else do we have to do?

HARRIS: You watch children in the playground and the little ones seem to know how to do this instinctively.

RESNICK: Our children don't need to be taught how to be happy, generally speaking. Children already know how to be happy. They know how to play. Children have a wonderful sense of humor right from the first. I've seen babies with a sense of humor; they make you laugh. What is playing peek-a-boo about? It's about a baby who doesn't have words, doing things to make you laugh, and they laugh, too.

LAUGH

"Children already know how to be happy. I've seen babies with a sense of humor; they make you laugh."

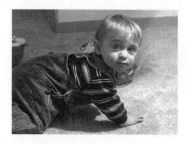

Children have a sense already of what happiness is. We de-condition it when we tell them, 'Stop being so exuberant, stop playing. Can't you do something productive? Sit still, stop fidgeting.' In many, many ways, we train children not to be happy. We also build in a certain amount of insecurity in children, because we tell them that there's a right way and a wrong way, and when they're doing it wrong, rather than reinforcing what they're doing right. What's most important is encouragement. We need to encourage children. We need to comfort children when they are afraid. We need to say to them, 'Yes, I understand that you're afraid, let me hug you, let me hold you. You're going to be okay, everything's going to be okay.' We can't deny their fears, because there are things to fear, and there is danger, and children need to know that. But we need to support them and comfort them. People who have never been comforted go through life fearful all the time. We need to give them a lot of love and, of course, all of this happens from birth on. Children learn from their parents. If the parent is fearful, if the parent gives himself or herself a hard time, if the

HUMOR

Enlighten up!

In 1964, *Saturday Review* editor Norman Cousins was told that he had a degenerative spinal condition, with a one-in-500 chance of surviving. In a story that has since become famous, Cousins began treating his condition with intensive doses of vitamins—and laughter: Marx Brothers movies, old episodes of *Candid Camera*, selections from humor anthologies. "It worked," he reported later, after discovering that 10 minutes of belly laughs provided him with at least two hours of pain-free sleep.

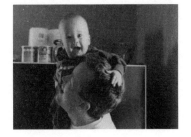

More recent studies offer additional evidence that humor, optimism, pleasure, and well-being are strong indicators of future good health. Researchers in Heidelberg, Germany, administered several tests to 3,440 residents in 1973 to determine the degree to which they were satisfied with life. Participants were selected for age only; anyone with major chronic disease was excluded. A follow-up study 21 years later found that 75 percent of the 300 highest scorers—those who described themselves as happiest—were alive and well, while only 2.5 percent of the 200 lowest scorers were still living.

parent is wounded, children are going to pick that up. There's no way, really, we can shield children from fear and pain and unhappiness. What we have to be able to do is help them deal with that, so that they become competent at living a pleasured, energetic, inspired life.

HARRIS: What do you most want us to remember about how to be happy?

RESNICK: More than anything else we really need to lighten up, and know that nothing is as bad as it seems. All we need to do, sometimes, is just change our way of looking at something. Sometimes a terrible disaster can become a wonderful opportunity for something new to happen. Lighten up, and let your spirit soar.

9 MINDFUL EATING

Have you ever looked up halfway through a party-sized bag of popcorn, your fingertips coated with cheese flavoring, only to realize that despite having no clear memory of what you'd consumed, your stomach was starting to protest that it was full while your mind still wanted more?

Maybe that's never been your experience, but it has been mine. As you make your way through this chapter, you may find yourself in there as readily as I did. As I went back over the interview with Geneen Roth, in fact, I realized how often I'm still guilty of using food as nothing more than fuel, something to be consumed at my desk while reading or working at the computer or (between mouthfuls) catching up on the phone calls I need to return.

For me, as for most of us, the habit of "oblivious eating" began in childhood. I couldn't get away with reading at the family dinner table, but any time I ate by myself, I always had a book in front of me. During the early years of my television career, things got worse. The pace of the news day was such that breakfast was whatever I could munch on while scanning the newspaper. Lunch was generally a hamburger consumed in one of the news vans, on the way to or from some assignment. When I started driving once a week from my anchor/reporter job in Charlotte, North Carolina, to cover the legislature in Raleigh, the WBTV station wagon quickly began to resemble a fast-food trash can. A bad day was when both lunch and dinner were eaten in the car. A *really* bad day was when lunch, dinner, and lunch the following day were all devoured on the road, and breakfast wasn't even a possibility. Years later, when I began commuting on a semi-regular basis from my home in Boston to the *Nightline* offices in New York, I defined a bad day as one in which both lunch and dinner consisted of the cheese-and-cracker snack on the Pan Am shuttle.

So, clearly, I'm not the role model on this topic, although I'm happy to say that my eating habits have improved, over time. I've grown to love spinach and broccoli, no doubt to the great astonishment of my mother. I find that I prefer fish and chicken and fresh fruits and salads, mostly because I have more energy and feel better when that's what I eat. I've also discovered that my body seems to work better when I drink water all day long. All of these ideas, of course, are things I encountered years ago, both at home, and in biology and home economics classes back in high school. I just wasn't listening then.

I wish I could tell you that now I eat mindfully every day, and that I truly savor every bite that goes into my mouth. Sorry. Not yet—but I am working on it. Anti-diet expert Geneen Roth is right: whether you're dealing with a health-threatening weight problem, or just want to appreciate the pleasure that good food can bring, mindful eating does take practice. She's also right that it's worth doing.

GENEEN ROTH

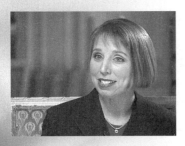

Geneen Roth learned the hard way about how to eat. Over a 17-year period that began when she was 11, she gained and lost over 1,000 pounds. It's a mind-boggling figure, especially to anyone who looks at her today, slim and glowing with good health. The author of *When You Eat at the Refrigerator, Pull Up A Chair*; *When Food is Love*; and *Feeding the Hungry Heart*, Roth also conducts anti-dieting workshops across the country.

HARRIS: You say that you started your first diet when you were 11 years old. How can that be?

ROTH: I wasn't fat, but everybody around me thought I should go on a diet, and so I did. I think my mother was concerned that I was going to follow in her footsteps. She had been fat her whole life, and it had caused her so much pain that she didn't want to see me following in that path. So I lost weight. My family doctor was happy, and my family was happy. Then I felt like, 'Oh, I can lose weight cutting out two pieces of bread and eating peaches instead of cookies. I bet I could even lose more weight if I did more radical things.'

So I started a 17-year course of very radical, crazy kinds of diets. I went on the prunes and meatball diet; I went on the hard-boiled egg, spinach and grapefruit diet; the one hot-fudge sundae a day diet; the fried-chicken diet. Even the 1,000-calorie-a-day sugar diet. I went on Atkins and Stillman's. When I was 15, I discovered diet pills. I stayed on those for four years without realizing that I was addicted to amphetamines. Went off of those at 19 and still kept going on more diets. Finally when I was 25, after going to India and learning about fasting, I decided I would become anorexic. Well, actually I didn't decide I was going to become anorexic, I decided I was going to be thin forevermore. I was never going to worry about being fat again.

HARRIS: No matter what.

ROTH: No matter what. Because it seemed to me at that point that every problem I had in my life could be traced back to the size of my body, and if only I were thin, then I would be happy. Or if only I were thin, then I would feel good enough about myself to do the things I needed to do in order to be happy.

It seemed to me that if I could be thin, then the entire rest of my life would fall into place. So I pretty much stopped eating. I ate 150 calories a day, jogged four miles a day, got down to 82 pounds, stayed that way for a year and a half, and still looked at myself and saw fat. Too round a face, too thick of thighs, arms that seemed kind of wavy. I just never looked at myself and saw thin.

Well, I couldn't stay at that weight because it wasn't my natural weight. After about a year and a half, I went on a binge. I do say that the fourth law of the universe is that for every diet, there's an equal and opposite binge. So I went on a binge to match that diet and I gained 80 pounds in two months.

HARRIS: Doing what? How could you possibly gain 80 pounds in two months?

ROTH: By never stopping the act of eating. I was eating at every moment of the day, cheesecake and ice cream, and everything I had deprived myself of. The only time I stopped eating was when I went to sleep. If I woke up in the middle of the night—straight to the refrigerator.

At the end of that period, I weighed 160 pounds, three months after I had weighed 82 pounds. I decided, both out of pain and out of some wisdom, that I had to do something. For 17 years, every single day, my life had revolved around what I ate, what I wanted to eat, the size of my body, what my life was going to be like when I got thin. At that point, I really believed that who I was, was what I weighed, that the two were synonymous. I felt like there had to be

MISERABLE

"For 17 years, every single day, my life had revolved around what I ate, what I wanted to eat, what my life was going to be like when I got thin, the size of my body...I knew I was killing myself in a very slow but very profound way. On top of that, I was miserable all of the time."

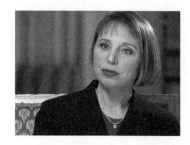

something more; I couldn't keep doing this. I knew I was killing myself in a very slow but very profound way. On top of that, I was miserable all of the time.

HARRIS: Ah, but were you happy when you were thin?

ROTH: No.

HARRIS: And being happy was the real goal, right?

ROTH: Yes, and I wasn't. So I started eating what I wanted to eat, and decided that I would never go on another diet again. I must say that that was one of the most terrifying things I've ever done, because I didn't trust myself. My lack of trust was in who I was and what I wanted, and what I believed and what I felt, and therefore in what I would eat if I let myself eat. What I have since learned is that how we feel about food, how we treat ourselves in the whole area of food and nourishment, is how we feel about ourselves in the rest of our lives. Whether we feel like we deserve to have what we want, whether we deserve to give ourselves pleasure, whether we deserve to have joy, whether it's okay to have abundance, what happens when we're surrounded by good things. Well, most people who've been on diets their whole lives feel like they'll destroy themselves if they eat what they want. They'll start eating at one end of their kitchen and chomp their way clear across the United States; they'll never stop. There's such a lack of trust and belief. And I saw that that's where I needed to spend my time and energy.

HARRIS: Where do you think this notion comes from, that food equals goodness or badness. 'Oh, I was bad last night, I had two pieces of chocolate cake.' What does eating have to do with being good or bad?

ROTH: I think it's a way of feeling like we're in control of our world. There's so much that happens that we're not in control of. Somehow we feel that if only we can get our food under control and we can be good, then somehow the uni-

"What I have since learned is that how we feel about food, how we treat ourselves in the whole area of food and nourishment, is how we feel about ourselves in the rest of our lives."

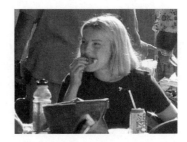

verse will be predictable. I'll tell you a story of somebody that I worked with in Seattle a few weeks ago. She stood up in a workshop and she said, 'I don't like anything I eat. I don't know what to eat. I feel bad every time I eat something good. I feel like somehow it's not okay to eat what I want, and I don't like the things that I'm supposed to eat that are good for me.' When I questioned her a little bit more, she said, 'I love living in Seattle, I love it here, and I love the man I'm about to marry. But I feel like that's enough goodness and that's enough pleasure in my life. Somehow it feels that if I don't like food, and if I deprive myself of food, then I won't have to pay for having this much pleasure here. I'll get to be in pain about this, I'll get to have what I can't live without, but basically I have to pay for the pleasure in my life. And I might as well pay for it by not liking what I eat.' It wasn't a conscious thing, it's not that she was aware that she was doing this, it was just that in the process of me being curious about it and asking her about it, she thought, 'Oh my goodness, I feel like I need to deprive myself of food, otherwise the things that I love in my life will get taken away from me.'

HARRIS: In other words, I'm only allowed this much happiness. I can't go the full spectrum. I can't have everything in my life be happy.

ROTH: No. And if we're not allowed to have it all, let me choose what I'll give up.

HARRIS: You encourage people to be curious about what they eat and how they eat. Why is that important?

ROTH: We believe so many things about food. First of all, most people believe that if they ate what they wanted to eat, they'd only eat sugar and fat in various combinations. They'd eat everything they are not supposed to or not allowed to eat. They'd eat everything that's not good for them. It's actually not

"Most people believe that if they ate what they wanted to eat, they'd only eat sugar and fat in various combinations. They'd eat everything they are not supposed to or not allowed to eat. They'd eat everything that's not good for them. It's actually not true."

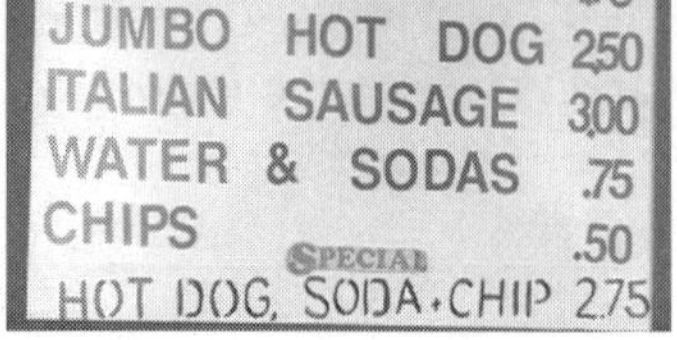

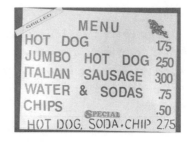

Angela Simms

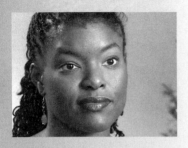

LIFE

Angela Simms remembers vividly the first time she became self-conscious about how much she weighed. At age five or six, her mother said, "Let's take a picture of you and send it to grandma, so she can see how fat you've gotten." It was a casual comment, made in jest, but it stuck with her. "From then on," she recalls, "I was the fat kid."

As she grew older, Angela remembers coming home after school to an empty house and eating and eating—"like a caged animal," she says—until someone else arrived. By her senior year in high school, she weighed in at 205 pounds.

In college, she majored in psychology and learned to recognize eating disorders. But knowing what they were didn't prevent her from acquiring one. Her problem began, ironically enough, after she had discovered exercise and lost 60 pounds. As friends told her how wonderful she looked, Angela started to worry about what would happen if she put the weight back on. Before she knew it, she was on the relentless cycle of bingeing and purging known as bulimia. By then, she was enrolled in nursing school. She knew how unhealthy her habit was, but was too ashamed of her painful secret to tell anyone. An irregular heartbeat and palpitations finally sent her to the doctor, who told her she might have to be on medication for the rest of her life.

Her next stop was at an anti-diet group known as Overcoming Overeating. Its philosophy is simple: diets don't work. There are no "forbidden" foods. Eat what you want, in moderation; if you deprive yourself, you'll only want it more. And if you're overeating, it's probably because of something else in your life, and you'd better figure out what it is.

In her new life as an overnight nurse at the Lakeland Regional Medical Center in Florida, Angela has devised several strategies to keep her eating under control. She carries a "food bag" with her at all times, usually filled with leftovers from something she's cooked at home. That way, she's never stuck somewhere hungry, with only high-fat, high-calorie choices. She avoids fast food and tries to stay away from the "thank-you" treats that families of patients bring in to the nursing staff, but she's also careful not to deprive herself.

"When I want a cookie," Angela says, "I eat one. I tell myself it's not going to become extinct overnight. I can have more tomorrow if I want it, and that keeps me from eating 20 of them.

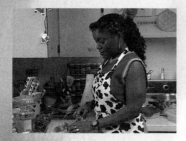 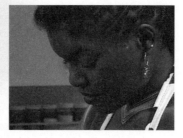 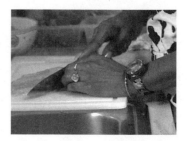

"On a day-to-day basis, you've got to listen to what your body wants. If you want ice cream for breakfast, have it. But if you find yourself eating gallons of ice cream for every meal, something's wrong. You need to ask yourself, 'Is there a problem?' If you're overeating, is it because you're depressed?"

At this point in her life, Angela can't guarantee she'll never have a problem with food again, but now she has a secret weapon: awareness.

"You've got to know yourself and listen to yourself. When that little warning bell goes off in your head, if you recognize it—that's half the battle."

true. When people start giving themselves permission—and this is a very scary thing to do for somebody who's been on a diet her whole life or his whole life, and believes that they're not to be trusted—when you say to yourself, 'How can I eat in a way that's going to enliven me, that's going to give me energy, that's going to let me do exactly what I want to do, that's going to let me be who I most want to be? How can I eat that way, instead of in a way that depresses me, that drains me, so when I roll over to one side of the bed, my stomach stays on the other side of the bed? How can I eat in a way where I'm not always focused on my stomach and my body and how I'm feeling tired—how can I eat that way?' When I start asking people that, they know intuitively what to eat. What most people don't know is that they can eat that way. They also don't know that it's okay to feel great, that you can eat foods that allow you to feel good.

There is so much terror around food, so much 'good' food and 'bad' food, and so much a feeling of, 'Ooh, I really want to be bad. And so let me be bad and break out and have everything I want. I'll just go straight to the Snickers, I'll go straight to the potato chips, I'll just go straight for something that's going to make me feel bad, because I want to be bad somehow. I want to break out.' I had somebody recently at the workshop, saying,'I just want to be bad, and the way that I'm expressing this badness is that I get to steal food somehow from my husband, or I steal it from my kids.' And I said, 'Well, what would you do if you would just let yourself be bad?' She said, 'I'd belt out a song, or I would just let myself be big and have a lot of energy.'

We translate all the issues in our lives through food. Food is like a microcosm. We use it to express our dreams, our fantasies, what we want to do, what we want to be. But the problem is that it keeps us wrapped around food and we don't look at the rest of our lives, because we're so worried about the size of our bodies that we never get to what we really want.

HARRIS: It sounds almost as if there's a little kid inside who's saying, 'I'm a grownup now, and I can eat all the chocolate chip cookies that I want.'

ROTH: And, 'You're not going to stop me.' So there's that rebellion there. But also what I'm teaching people more and more is how to be in touch with what they most want. What do you really want? Yes, I know that those candies look good and those doughnuts look good, but how are you going to feel after you eat them? When I say, 'Eat what you want to eat, stop when you've had enough, but learn to eat in a way that gives you energy, that allows you to feel awake and alive and fabulous,' then that changes it a little bit for people.

HARRIS: A lot of that involves the process coming to be known as mindful eating, being aware of what you're eating.

ROTH: Yes.

HARRIS: Why does that make a difference?

ROTH: Because when you eat something, you can tell almost immediately whether it makes you tired, sleepy, sick, or whether it gives you energy. You can tell after you finish eating how you feel. There's the sense of being aware and focused on tasting in the classes that I teach. We do some hands-on exercises with food, with a potato chip and a raisin and a chocolate kiss. People spend time eating each of these things. Now, most people are used to eating fistfuls of raisins, and bags of chips, and 20 chocolate kisses at a time. When they spend time touching, tasting, and allowing themselves to have what they have, then what happens is what happened a few days ago when I was teaching.

Somebody said, 'You know, I've eaten bags of chocolate kisses but I've never tasted one, and when I taste one, one is enough.'

So the mindfulness involved in eating allows you to be present. I encourage people to be present, not just with food, but with their lives. That means if you're eating, eat. Be right there with the food. Notice how it tastes. Notice how it feels in your mouth. Somebody said, 'You know, I thought I loved chocolate, but this feels kind of gummy in my mouth. I actually don't want another one, and I would have been reaching for the next one before I tasted this one.'

That's how most of us live the rest of our lives. We're in the present, but we're thinking about the past, or we're thinking about the future, what we don't have, what we want to have, what will make us happy. We never see what is it we have right now.

HARRIS: You carry around a bar of chocolate for that reason.

ROTH: I carry a chunk of chocolate everywhere because I like chocolate, but I know how much I can eat before I start feeling sick. I love the taste of it, and I found that if I focused just on the taste of one piece of chocolate, I could really let myself enjoy it. The thing is, most people feel so much guilt about food that when they're eating chocolate, they're going, 'I shouldn't be eating this, this is too fattening, this has X grams of fat, I'm going to have to pay for this later.' And then they've missed the whole thing. It's like visiting with a friend while you're talking on the phone and watching television. The friend comes in, you're watching television, she's there for 15 minutes, even an hour, you've been talking on the phone the whole time, she leaves and you feel like I never had the visit with my friend. That's what most of us do with food. We're eating but we're watching television, we're reading, we're driving in the car, and we're not focused on the food. Sometimes I say to people, 'Why do you eat in the car?' 'Well, nobody can see me in the car.' And I'll say, 'Well, now, let's see. You're in a vehicle surrounded by windows, everybody else is in a vehicle surrounded by windows, but nobody can see you?' 'But nobody I know can see me.' And then the question becomes, 'What would happen if somebody you knew saw what you ate?' 'They wouldn't love me.' So then, again—and this is why food is so fascinating—what I see is that the message is: 'If they saw me, they wouldn't love me. Who I am cannot be seen.' Again, this gets played out with food.

Ronna Kabatznick

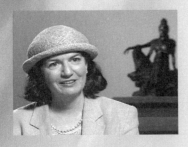

Despite a Ph.D. in psychology and nine years of working with Weight Watchers on their psychological approach to weight loss, it was as a volunteer at a soup kitchen that Ronna Kabatznick made the discovery that "eating is a source of delight, not a source of misery." On the basis of that revelation, she founded a national organization called Dieters Feed the Hungry—enabling those with too much food in their lives to help those with too little, thereby nourishing both groups.

The program flourished, until a firestorm ripped through the hills of Oakland and burned 3,000 homes to the ground, including her own. All her work—including the resource files for Dieters Feed the Hungry—went up in flames, leaving her with only the clothes she was wearing. Shortly thereafter, she suffered the loss of her brother, father, grandmother, and a close friend, one after the other. Then she became so ill that she was forced to stop working for a time.

Stripped of three cherished family members, a lifetime of possessions, and, for a time, her sense of identity as a psychologist, Kabatznick immersed herself in the principles of Buddhism, as she questioned how to find balance in the midst of change, and peace in the midst of suffering.

In her book, *The Zen of Eating: Ancient Answers to Modern Weight Problems,* she suggests that peace and security cannot be found by being a certain weight or being able to fit into a particular outfit. Instead, Kabatznick believes, emotional hunger grows deeper and more painful the more you struggle against it, while suffering ends by letting go of attachment to things that can't offer true nourishment.

"The key to healthy eating is learning how to change your state of mind," Kabatznick says. "What you eat or don't eat isn't nearly as important."

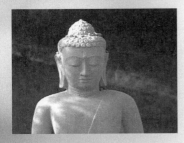
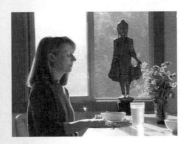
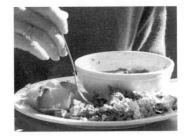

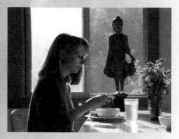 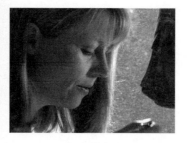 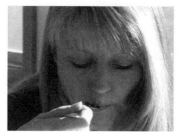

When asked her advice on how to lose weight and keep it off, Kabatznick used to suggest things like regular exercise or eating a variety of foods in moderation. These days, she strongly recommends a daily meditation or mindfulness practice, instead.

"I only suggest practicing the recipes for nourishing the heart. Food for the heart provides the only kind of nourishment that lasts. Be mindful, be kind, be generous, be grateful, and learn to let things be."

HARRIS: So in some sense it's really not about food. It's about nourishment, it's about love, it's about a lot of inner conversations going on.

ROTH: Yes. It's about all that. It's about food, too, and that's why food is such a beautiful path inside. There's actual physical food that you're eating that evokes a particular physical effect, a biochemical effect in you, but how you feel about food and how you feel about yourself is all connected. So when somebody feels as if they can't be seen and who they are is not lovable—that if they let themselves have what they wanted, people around them would be disgusted or would turn away—that has much more to do with inner feelings of self than it has to do with food. But it all gets played out through food, because how could it not? It's you doing it, so if you feel that way about yourself, it's going to be reflected in whatever you do.

HARRIS: How do you get people to take that leap from, 'I'm fat, I'm ugly, nobody cares about me,' to, 'Whatever size I am, I'm pretty terrific right now.'

ROTH: One thing that I'm teaching people to do is to come back in their bodies. Most of us live in our minds. We are comparing ourselves all the time to what we think we should look like, or what somebody else has told us we need to look like. We hardly ever spend time in our bodies. By that, I mean sensing our legs, sensing our arms, feeling that we exist in this body. The mind can drive you insane. There's no end to what the mind tells you you should look like. It keeps telling you, 'When you have this, you will be happy.' Oftentimes in a workshop I'll say to 500 people, 'How many of you have lost weight before?' Everybody raises their hands. 'How many of you were ecstatically happy when you lost weight before?' Four people raise their hands. 'How many of you believe you will be ecstatically happy when you lose weight again?'

HARRIS: Everybody.

ROTH: Everybody raises their hands. And I think, what's that about? So a lot of my work is directed to helping people see what they believe that's actually not true. It's not true, and they already know it's not true, but they are not act-ing on what they know. So that's part of it. The other thing I have people do is stay in their bodies. Begin to feel what living in this body feels like. In this moment, there's usually not a lot wrong. Yes, they're not the size they want to be, but just sensing their arms and being grateful for the fact that we have arms, that we have legs, that we can move, that we have a body. Part of it is just being here, with this body, now.

Another thing is living as if you already like yourself. Live as if you are, already, who you think you need to be, for you to like yourself. That means when you wake up in the morning, you live as if you already like yourself. What would that look like, how would you dress, how would you walk, what would you eat?

Another thing that I spend time working with is helping people identify and disengage from what I call the 'fat and ugly attack voice.' Everybody's got that voice. Everybody's got the voice that says, 'You're not doing it right, you're not okay.' The voice goes something like, 'I can't believe you just did that, I can't believe you just ate that. I can't believe you are who you are—what's the matter with you?' Everybody's got that. Most of us believe it, and most of us collapse under it. That voice just comes in and takes over, kind of usurps a person's mind. It's like they've got this alien inside.

So I help people disengage from that. When that voice comes in and says, 'I can't believe you're eating that for lunch,' I teach people to either brush it off, or deal with it with humor, saying, 'Yeah, and you should have seen what I ate for breakfast!' Or, 'You're not my friend, and you're not allowed to talk to me like that.' People have to disengage from that voice, because that voice runs our lives, and for any change to happen we need to disengage.

HARRIS: I want to ask you about the common ways in which we all delude ourselves about what we're eating. For example, when you stand in front of the refrigerator, you could be ingesting a lot of calories—but those don't count, right? Because you're not really eating, you're just kind of checking it out.

ROTH: That's right. Americans open the refrigerator door 33 times a day. When you think about it, you look, and then 10 minutes later you look again, and then a half hour later you look again, just to see if the contents have shifted since the last time you looked, or in case somebody's added something. Most of us swing by the refrigerator on our way to the phone, or on our way to the bedroom, even on our way to the bathroom. We stand there grazing around, picking at food with our fingers, but we're not really eating, we're just on the way somewhere else. What I say is, would you ask a friend to come over to dinner, tell them, 'We're going to eat the way I eat, come on in,' then go to the refrigerator, open the door, she's looking at you like, 'Where's the table, where's the silverware, where are the plates?' 'Nope, no table, no silverware, no plates, finger time.' And you give her a Tupperware container, and then you give her yesterday's Chinese food, and then you pull out the ice cream and, yes, even with the ice cream, we're going to be using our fingers to get that soft little melting spot around the edges. That's how most of us treat ourselves with food.

So there's not the awareness that we're eating. There's also not any enjoyment because as you're standing there at the refrigerator eating, you're not enjoying what you're doing. You're thinking, 'I'm just getting this in my mouth before I can get on to the next thing.' A lot of the other ways that people do that is: broken cookies don't count, because when the cookie breaks the calories break, or frozen food that's still frozen doesn't count, or edging a cake when the cake is a little uneven and you just have to even it out on the side; or free food, food at a supermarket, birthdays, anniversaries, celebrations, vacations, if you're sick…

HARRIS: …anything on your child's plate…

ROTH: Anything on your child's plate. Those kinds of things. Or if somebody gives it to you. Somebody recently said to me, 'You know, when somebody gives me a gift of food, I feel like I need to eat it because I want the love. I feel like if I don't eat the food, then somehow I'll be rejecting the love, and who am I to reject love given to me.' So, really, it's that edge between food and everything else, between food and love and pleasure and compassion and abundance and patience. All of those things are related, very much related—food and love.

HARRIS: How do you manage to keep it in some kind of balance, then? Are there ten rules for mindful eating or seven rules for mindful eating? Or just, 'Pay attention to what you're eating'—does that do it?

ROTH: In the beginning, it takes a lot of awareness and it takes a commitment to the process. People have to be willing to be mindful about what they're eating. To eat when they're hungry, to be aware of what hunger feels like. A lot of people can't even remember the last time they got hungry, or they eat for the hunger to come. They're storing up all the time for the next time they might get hungry, as if we don't have all these convenience stores everywhere around us, and we can't stop every 15 minutes for food. So, eat when you're hungry is one of them, and eat sitting down in a calm environment. This doesn't include the car, it doesn't include reading and eating. Eat what you want. That's what your body wants, and, of course, it's not what your mind wants. Your mind can go insane with what it wants: 'I want what that person is eating and I want what I saw in the store yesterday.' It's really, 'What does my body want right now?' Eat until you've had enough. Satisfaction is both emotional and physical. There's a physical point of satisfaction. It happens often that somebody is eating, and then there's one point at which your body says, 'I've had enough now, anything you put inside me is for your mind, not for me, your body.' You've got to be paying attention there, so that means you've got to be present. If you're distracted, if you're doing something else, you're going to miss that signal.

It's a practice. Most of us are not used to paying attention. We eat because it's breakfast, lunch, or dinner time, or because someone puts it in front of us, or because we're at a restaurant or at a supermarket and it's free. The basic guideline is: when you eat, eat. When you do other things, do other things. Recently I've been recommending to people that when they sit down, they take just a moment to realize that they're sitting down and give some kind of thanks that

H U N G E R

"People have to be willing to be mindful about what they're eating. To eat when they're hungry, to be aware of what hunger feels like. A lot of people can't even remember the last time they got hungry, or they eat for the hunger to come."

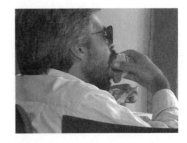

there's food on the table. That they're sitting, either by themselves or with people that they like or love, friends, companions, co-workers. Just take a moment. From running around to sitting at the table and then just digging right in, there needs to be some kind of transition: 'Oh, there's food here, we're eating now, let me pay attention and also be grateful that there's food on the table, and we have something to eat.' It's finding a balance somehow, eating food that you like that tastes good in your mouth, and being mindful while you're doing it.

HARRIS: And trusting your body to know when it's had enough.

ROTH: Yes.

HARRIS: Is it important to remember that when you're eating, you're not 'just' eating, it's not just a physical act?

ROTH: Yes, it is really important, because it involves presence and showing up. But in order to have the eating be balanced in your mind, it's also important to have another kind of life, not just centered around food. What I encourage people to do is have balance in their non-food-related life. To have a life you can go to when you've had enough food. A lot of people say, 'But there's nothing as good as food.' There's a whole world as good as food. But, again, that takes practice. A part of what I recommend to people, and part of what I'm teaching, is that they have something that they do every day that allows them to center themselves, to be with themselves, to be inside their bodies. Usually, it's something quiet and alone. It could be just sitting for 15 minutes a day. If somebody doesn't have 15 minutes, then 10 minutes doing some kind of curiosity dialogue where they're asking themselves just a simple, open-ended question, 'Where am I now?' That allows you to start being interested and curious about yourself, and to start treating yourself with kindness, which is really important. Self-care and kindness, and the third factor: curiosity and the willingness to act on your own behalf. To see that if you need time alone, you take

B A S I C

"The basic guideline is when you eat, eat. When you do other things, do other things."

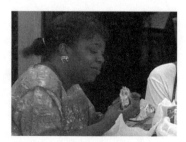

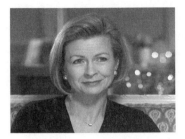 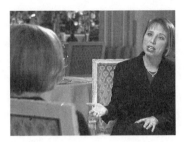 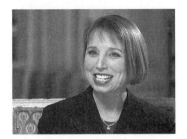

five minutes, even if you're at work and it means going to the bathroom and sitting in a bathroom stall for five minutes. Just taking time alone, going outside and breathing, being willing to do what you need to do to care for yourself.

HARRIS: I was just about to ask whether you think obsession with food goes with unhappiness in other areas of your life. In other words, is it possible to be a happy person in every other aspect of your life, but still be very unhappy about food?

ROTH: I don't think so. If you feel that you deserve goodness and kindness and pleasure, if you feel that you deserve to take good care of yourself, then that's got to be reflected in how you eat. I don't think it's possible to be happy and to hate your body, to be constantly judging your body and want to be thinner, even 10 pounds thinner and have this constant litany of, 'I'm not good enough, I'm not thin enough, I need to lose 10 pounds.' To be happy in every area of life, it's all part of the same fabric, all a part of a whole here. What I'm talking about is having people feel what it's like, to understand that in this moment, there's nothing wrong. Everything's okay.

HARRIS: What, if anything, does this have to do with getting in touch with your spiritual side?

ROTH: In some ways, it has everything to do with it. People come to me because they feel that there is something wrong with their lives, and that if they lost weight, whatever's wrong with their lives would be right. Even though usually these very same people have lost weight two, three, four, ten times—and whatever's wrong with their lives was still wrong when they lost weight. What all this has to do with is getting in touch with what you eat as a way to nourish yourself and allow you to be all you can be. It has to do with opening your heart. It has to do with learning how to live the life that you're living in a way that you want most to live it, and what that takes is practice. It's not just, 'Oh, all right, fine, I'll write down three things I'm grateful for every night, and then everything will be fine.' That's a way in; that's a practice. But it's understanding that food isn't the end to all of this, that losing weight is not the end, that there's joy and compassion and wisdom. That there's a way to tap into those things in yourself, that each of us is so much greater than we ever imagined we could be. To tap into that takes some kind of practice you do every day. A mindfulness practice, a sitting practice, takes becoming aware of your reactions to things. It takes knowing yourself. What you eat and how you eat and when you eat also takes knowing yourself. Mindfulness with food is a skill you develop, and as you become more mindful with food, it's a skill that can translate to other areas of your life.

HARRIS: We've been talking a lot about attitudes towards food, some of them peculiar and some of them a more balanced way to think about it. I'm wondering whether you also believe that we have a responsibility to our bodies to nourish them properly.

ROTH: What I believe is that everybody's got a job description. By that, I mean we all are here to be doing something in particular. Each of us is unique, each of us has different talents, each of us is good at different things. I know my job description is writing books and teaching, and what I feel like I need to do is eat in a way that supports me in doing what my job is this time. The purpose of mindful eating is not just to be conscious and to be aware and to be present, although that's all part of it. That is, in itself, incredibly satisfying and fulfilling, and also allows you to have a very deep intimacy with yourself. The benefit of that is that it allows you to have the energy to go figure out what your job description is and then to do it.

We're on the earth to do something, to give something. It doesn't have to be about writing books or being on television. It could be being the best mother, or the best father. It could be being the best cook, or the best waitress, or the best bank teller that you can be. Everybody knows they're doing their job description when what they're doing makes their heart sing. Eating corresponds to that, in the sense that when you eat in a way that deeply nourishes your body, then you're able to do what you're meant to do in the fullest and most exhilarating way that you can.

10 EAST/WEST MEDICINE

Pity the poor physician trying to practice medicine in America today. After years of Herculean effort preparing for, slogging through, and finally graduating from medical school, with the triple challenges of managed care, malpractice worries, and staggering student loans, no wonder so many doctors are beginning to wonder why they chose the career they did.

Now, there is a new urgency to the question. It was front-page news across the country in November of 1998 when a study published in the *Journal of the American Medical Association* showed that Americans paid more visits to alternative care practitioners in the previous year than to their primary care physicians. What began 10 years ago as a murmur from the masses has grown into a full-throated roar of discontent from consumers, who complain that traditional Western medicine is expensive, unresponsive, and uncaring. They want something else—and if necessary, are willing to pay for it out of their own pockets.

Not surprisingly, perhaps, it is baby boomers leading the charge. I say 'not surprisingly,' because many, if not most of us, have been questioning conventional wisdom all our lives. Whether or not we smoked marijuana or experimented with other drugs in the '60s, we prefer not to take drugs now. We see how our parents are aging, and make fierce vows that we won't follow in their footsteps. We intend to look as young as possible and remain healthy and vigorous forever—or at least for as long as we possibly can.

With patients like us, what's a physician to do? Faced with demands for information about acupuncture, massage therapy, herbs and vitamins, anti-aging strategies, homeopathy, naturopathy—it isn't surprising that many doctors might react with alarm and apprehension. After all, these weren't topics covered in the curriculums of most medical schools. Investigating and then incorporating the best of the complementary therapies is surely not easy, especially while trying to maintain a busy medical practice.

It may not be easy, but it is happening. Across the country, thousands of doctors now offer a holistic menu of choices: everything from acupuncture and nutrition counseling to Reiki and yoga. If the polls are right—like the recent one from *Time*/CNN showing that 84 percent of Americans who visited an alternative practitioner said they would do so again—it is these doctors whose practices will continue to thrive, well into the next century.

What's happening represents a virtual tidal wave of change, for patients as well as doctors. As health-conscious consumers, we have been inundated with information for years, and it's beginning to sink in. We know more than we ever have about what's required to keep our bodies in good health; what's more, we are increasingly willing to accept that responsibility. The old way was to assume that it was the doctor's job to fix us when we were "broken," much as we handed over the keys to the auto mechanic when the car needed repair. The new way is to be attentive to our minds and bodies all the time; to draw on ancient wisdom along with the latest research, as we learn to stimulate our innate ability to heal; to make informed choices across the board, in a genuine partnership with our healthcare provider. Whether we visit a doctor of medicine or a doctor of naturopathy, a cardiologist or a chiropractor, the maintenance of our good health is up to us at least as much as it is up to them.

Change is not only coming; it's here. Centuries-old ideas from the East are merging more and more with technology and training from the West. Each can learn much from the other. As what was once "alternative" now becomes mainstream, it's my hope that physicians and patients alike can approach this brave new world with their minds—and hearts—wide open to the possibilities.

STEPHEN SINATRA

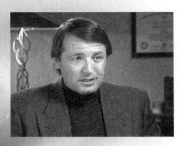

For the past two decades, Stephen Sinatra, M.D., has been utilizing nutritional, psychological, and other complementary therapies along with conventional treatments in his practice in Manchester, Connecticut. He is a board-certified cardiologist and certified bioenergetic analyst, with more than 10 years of postgraduate training in the crucial role that behavior and emotion play in heart disease. Sinatra is the author of *Heartbreak & Heart Disease: A Mind/Body Prescription for Healing the Heart; Optimum Health;* and *Lose to Win: A Cardiologist's Guide to Weight Loss.*

HARRIS: As you look back on medical school, is there anything about what you were taught there that doesn't square with your view of the world now?

SINATRA: First of all, medical school is an unbelievable experience. It's like studying for college finals every three days, because there are so many disciplines that you learn. But when you go out into the real world, there's a lot that was missing. For example, I'm very big into nutrition and mind/body medicine and emotional healing. None of that was taught in medical school. In nutritional healing alone, I had maybe one lecture in four years. When I look at the world now, I see a whole paradigm shift. Medical school needs to train a doctor not only in conventional medicine but also in preventive medicine. Preventive medicine is really the whole key to staying healthy and being well and aging gracefully.

HARRIS: What are we learning, particularly from complementary therapies, about how we can stay healthy as opposed to trying to fix ourselves once there's a problem?

SINATRA: Well, that's sort of the old paradigm: you have a problem, you fix it. The new medicine is where the health practitioner will support his patient's body into doing the healing by itself. But there's a blend. I'll give you an example. If I had a heart attack, I would want the best board-certified cardiologist to do whatever he or she has to do to help me survive. After the heart attack, if I did survive, then get me to a naturopath, or preventive medical doctor, or somebody who can place me on a right road to healing. In other words, get me into lifestyle adjustments, which would include mind/body medicine, emotional healing, metabolic healing, vitamins and minerals, a healthy diet, exercise, meditation. All those lifestyle interventions would really nurture my heart, heal my heart, and prevent a subsequent heart attack.

HARRIS: Let's talk specifically about why those would make a difference. What's wrong with the way that doctors have been treating patients for years, not just for heart disease but a whole range of issues?

SINATRA: Well, it's simple. A person gets sick, they go to a doctor, and they want the cure. For example, let's say they have an infection. A doctor may give an antibiotic. But that's why we have so many resistant strains of bacteria today, because of all the over-zealous use of antibiotics. People want to be fixed, whether it's high blood pressure, 'Give me the pill for high blood pressure,' or, 'I'm overweight, give me a pill to lose weight.' But the body pays a tremendous price when you do these pharmaceutical interventions. If you look at the history of medicine, in the time of Hippocrates the dogma was, 'First, do no harm.' Since the discovery of penicillin in the late '30s, early '40s, the whole medical industry has become pharmaceutically oriented. That can have its advantages, but unfortunately many, many doctors have become prescription writers, and that's not where good medicine is today. It may be good for certain aspects of medicine, but it's not where real healing comes in.

HARRIS: A lot of doctors, many of them conventionally trained as you were, have turned to other techniques, other practices. What do you think is driving that?

"Many doctors have become prescription writers, and that's not where good medicine is today. It may be good for certain aspects of medicine, but it's not where the real healing comes in."

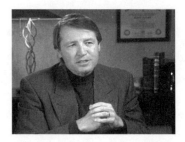

SINATRA: I think it's the public. People want a real, conventional medical doctor. There's no doubt about it. They want a doctor who has gone through the system, who is well trained in conventional medicine. But they also want a doctor who is open to all these complementary healing techniques: mind/body techniques, nutritional healing, vitamin and mineral therapies, all the different therapies we use to reduce stress. People want that. If a doctor isn't able to be flexible, then that doctor is going to be a dinosaur. The Achilles heel of the medical profession is our rigidity, our double-blind studies. Doctors forget that one patient with diabetes was given insulin in the 1920s and improved. There were no huge double-blind studies done on diabetes in the 1920s. It took one patient. Yet today we've become so scientifically oriented it's become our Achilles heel, and our rigidity is our downfall.

HARRIS: What should doctors be doing instead?

SINATRA: Listening to our patients. Our patients are our messengers. When a patient comes in and says to me, 'Dr. Sinatra, I heard that horse chestnut will help my inflamed veins.' If I don't know anything about horse chestnut, I'm not going to say, 'No, no, no, that's bogus.' I'll read about it, I'll look into that. What a good doctor today has to do is look at their patient and let them be a messenger. If they suggest alternative healing techniques, it's that doctor's job to look into these aspects to see if they have merit. That's what I've done with my patients over the years.

HARRIS: Are some doctors resistant to that idea?

SINATRA: Absolutely. There are doctors who will fire their patients if they take vitamins and minerals when they have heart disease. I mean, that's the rigidity I'm getting at. The best doctors are the ones who will use the best of conventional medicine and complement it. That's what their patients want, so that's what a good doctor will do. He or she will empower the patient, nurture that patient, give them more things to choose from in the healing process.

MESSENGER

"What a good doctor today has to do is look at their patient and let them be a messenger. If they suggest alternative healing techniques, it's that doctor's job to look into these aspects to see if they have merit."

HARRIS: If patient demand is driving some doctors to re-think how they practice medicine, what do you think is spurring that demand? What is it about how people think about their bodies that has changed?

SINATRA: More people today are taking responsibility for their health. There are so many things now in our environment that we have to look at preventive medicine. If we don't, we're going to perish. And this is where the baby boomer generation is driving this whole aspect of preventive medicine and anti-aging medicine—longevity medicine, I call it. Just think about this: if you could take a little vitamin C and vitamin E and other beta-carotenoids that can prevent macular degeneration or prevent cataracts in your eyes for an extra 10 years, that's wonderful. That's good preventive medicine, and that's just the tip of the iceberg. I could talk about heart disease, cancer, and nutritional supplements for a long time, and I haven't even touched on emotional release work, which is another factor in all these illnesses. Overall, people are taking more responsibility for themselves, and their physicians are empowering them to do that.

HARRIS: The good ones.

SINATRA: That's right, the good ones.

HARRIS: You've written that people can't afford to get sick in America. Why not?

SINATRA: You don't want to get sick in America today, because we have a managed care system. Who's going to control the case if you get sick? Is it the doctor, is it the health provider, is it the insurance company, is it some bureaucrat? People are finally grabbing the bull by the horns and are refusing to get sick. That's where I see the whole paradigm shift going in America today. People will be taking more responsibility for themselves, will be getting less involved with unhealthy habits, will be taking nutritional supplements, will be

I N S U R A N C E

"You don't want to get sick in America today, because we have a managed care system. Who's going to control the case if you get sick? Is it the doctor, is it the health provider, is it the insurance company, is it some bureaucrat? People are finally grabbing the bull by the horns and are refusing to get sick."

Libby Barnett and Maggie Chambers

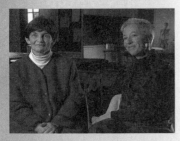

P R O F I L E

After a day of unseasonably hot temperatures for late spring, an early evening thunderstorm has finally cooled the second-floor classroom inside the old Watertown High School in suburban Boston—now home to the New England School of Acupuncture. A refreshing breeze lifts the faded yellow shades at the windows as it ripples through the room, sending a sigh of relief through the class of 20 Reiki students.

Reiki Masters Libby Barnett and Maggie Chambers stand in front of two plastic chairs as they continue their lecture and slide show on the history and application of this 2,500-year-old healing art. As they do, each places her hands on the shoulders of a volunteer, to offer a 10-minute sample treatment.

"I can't believe how warm her hands were," whispers one woman to her neighbor as she resumes her seat. "They were like heating pads."

"Could you feel anything?"

The first woman nods. "I don't know what it was, exactly, but there was definitely something."

Had they heard the exchange, Libby and Maggie would have smiled. They have been "feeling something" from Reiki (pronounced ray-kee) for decades. Libby, a former medical social worker at Massachusetts General Hospital, and Maggie, an artist and mother of four, conduct classes together at The Reiki Healing Connection in Wilton, New Hampshire, and at hospices, medical centers, and medical schools throughout the United States. Each achieved the level of Reiki Master after months of study and years of practice.

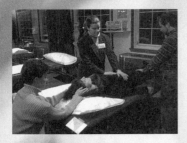
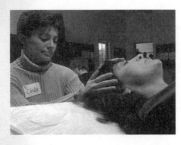
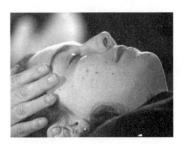

As they explain in their book, *Reiki: Energy Medicine*, Reiki is an ancient art of touch therapy from Tibet, rediscovered by a Japanese monk educator in the mid-1800s. Over the past 10 years, this once-obscure healing art has become increasingly accepted within more conventional settings in the West. In some medical practices, Reiki treatments are routinely recommended to surgical patients, both pre- and post-operatively.

"I became interested in Reiki back in the '70s because I had always wanted to offer something that patients could take home with them to augment their healing process," recalls Libby. "First I used it on myself, my children, and my husband, to help with injuries and upsets. It really caught my attention when nurses told me my son's broken wrist had healed in two-thirds the expected time. After seeing the difference it made in our family life, I began incorporating it into my work with my clients when appropriate. Now clients actively seek me out because they have heard that I combine Reiki with psychotherapy."

Maggie's first encounter with Reiki was after giving birth to her fourth child. "I was so exhausted after the exertion of childbirth, and it was remarkable how blissful I became after the treatment. I was excited at the thought of being able to use Reiki with my husband and children, and I've been utterly surprised and delighted with the depth of its contribution to my personal life. It has had a profoundly transformative effect."

Reiki Masters say the purpose of Reiki is to tap into the life energy that is part of all living things, thereby connecting universal energy with the body's innate powers of healing, and restoring balance on physical, mental, and emotional levels.

"The same biological intelligence that enables the body to heal a cut finger or mend a broken bone is amplified by Reiki," says Libby. "It's easy to learn and doesn't require complicated techniques, so health-

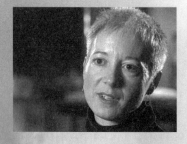
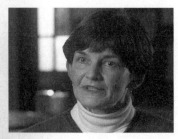

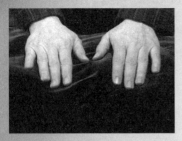 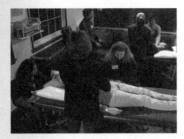 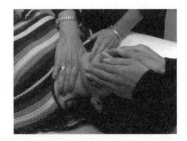

care practitioners of many disciplines are able to incorporate it easily into their specialties."

The vision of health care that Libby and Maggie hold for the future is one of partnership, rather than competition, with traditional medicine. "We can hold fast to the idea that encourages the use and development of technology and sophisticated procedures, increasingly able to fully service only the elite in our society. Or we can begin fashioning a healthcare system that provides services that are simple and inexpensive when they can be, and complex and expensive only when they must be."

taking time out for life, will be getting into their hearts, cultivating closer relationships and a little spirituality. What's going to happen is that disease is just going to go down.

HARRIS: Is it more satisfying for you as a physician to be addressing all of these other issues?

SINATRA: I love my work. When I can help put a patient on the right path, it's wonderful. But I have to make something clear. I'm not the doctor; all I am is the nurse. Nature heals. I don't heal anybody. All I can do is steer them into the right direction, empower them to get on the right path, and then miracles can happen. And, yes, it does give me a lot of satisfaction.

HARRIS: How did you first start learning about complementary therapies?

SINATRA: When I finished my cardiology training in 1977, just after the Vietnam War had come to a close, I saw a lot of sudden deaths in young men. It was frightening, because these were young men in their early '30s. They didn't smoke, they were athletes like I was, they ate a healthy diet, so I concluded it was all due to a lot of stress. As a cardiologist, I was working with this day and night, and what was absolutely horrifying was that it was like looking in the mirror. I mean, I had the same issues as these guys, so in 1977, I started to go into psychotherapy. I attended a two-year gestalt training program in Hartford, and then I went into a 10-year bioenergetic therapy training program in Boston and became a certified bioenergetic psychotherapist. It really opened me up to a whole range of other possiblities in good health.

HARRIS: What is bioenergetics?

SINATRA: Bioenergetics is the study of energy in one's body. I believe that it's blocked energy that causes illness. Let me give you an example. If you take stagnant water—over time, it becomes toxic. Or suppose you're stagnant in your bowels and you're constipated over and over again, that could predispose you to bowel cancer. Same thing occurs with heart disease or any other illness. If I'm not breathing properly, and I have stagnant energy in my chest, I can predispose myself to heart disease. A woman who has terrific anger and resentment in her upper body, who has this 'energy lock,' may predispose herself to breast cancer. So bioenergetics is a type of body–oriented therapy which enhances energy. In other words, if we have an energy block in the throat, we would use a lot of the voice to unblock it. If we have an energy block in the pelvis, we would use exercises in the pelvis to open up that energy, reduce the rigidity in the body and help cells pulsate. When cells pulsate, they're alive and healthy. When they become frozen or stagnant, when they become very contracted, whether that's due to stress or metabolics or environmental toxins, then we get illness. That's the essence of bioenergetics.

HARRIS: In fact, you've written that becoming ill, or 'dis-eased', as you put it, is a result of an imbalance of mind and body and spirit. Some of your physician colleagues would say, 'Where'd you get that?'

SINATRA: That's a good question. I believe that when we're out of balance with anything in our body, if we have intense anger and it's not released, it can cause high blood pressure. If we have incredible sadness and it's not released, it can cause heartbreak. And if you don't release the sadness, heartbreak can cause heart disease. When I became a trained psychotherapist, I looked at this whole mind/body aspect of medicine and embraced the idea that our emotional life is just as important as our physical life. And then there's a spiritual connection as well. Whenever you confront a person with an illness, you have to involve everything, including the spiritual. Let me give you an example. I've had corporate executives looking at the ceiling for four days after they've had a heart attack. They were in the cardiac care unit for four days. And some of them got it. They absolutely got it. They changed their life around, because when you have a life-threatening illness, you must look deeper into your spiritual or emotional self, and that's what some people will do. But some people don't get it. They'll just recreate the illness again when they leave the hospital. You have to involve all aspects of healing—the psychological, emotional, and spiritual—to help get people on the path to healing and wellness.

HARRIS: Do you think that the same people who are interested in complementary or alternative therapies are also more interested in spiritual aspects of their lives?

SINATRA: It's hard to say because people are different. One thing I do know, as a doctor, is that every person has an avenue to get to them. Let me give you an example. If I'm treating a Pratt & Whitney aeronautical engineer, and I start talking about spirituality, he's gone. But if I approach this engineer, and I start to talk about his heart attack, and diet and exercise and left-brain stuff, he'll connect with me. It's almost like a dance, where a patient begins to trust a healer. After you have this relationship, then you can tie in other stuff, like right-brain stuff. I may tell this engineer, 'Okay, we've changed your diet; I've put you on the vitamin and mineral program; we've got you into an exercise program.' After he begins to trust me, then I might say, 'Well, look, let's play a little bit. Why don't you try a little prayer or yoga, a little meditation or maybe some rolfing or Tai Chi.' You have to assess your patient and if they're very, very left-brain and you come in with a right-brain approach, they're gone. If they're right-brained, and you come in with the right-brain approach, they'll give you a hug and a kiss. But that's how you have to do this dance with patients. You must take your time because the healing process is a very difficult process. What patients want is two things: one, they want you to see their suffering, and two, you have to establish trust. What I really learned about being a psychoanalyst is that trust is so important. Medical doctors are no different.

HARRIS: One of the things you say you notice about your patients is how they breathe. Why is that important?

SINATRA: Have you ever seen people who breathe so fast it's like they're trying to suck up their breath? I call it chaotic breathing, and this is bad for the heart over time. There were studies in Poland, for example, that people who have chaotic, interrupted, non-pulsating breathing get more heart disease. Now, what is healthy breathing? It's very simple. It's like diaphragmatic breathing, where we can put our hands on our belly, breathe through our nose and exhale through our mouth, where we're lifting up our abdomen and we take a deep

Susan Goldberg

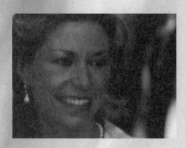

LIFE

At first glance, Susan Goldberg might seem an unusual enthusiast about the benefits of acupuncture. A nurse anesthetist, she is married to a vascular surgeon; her training and experience all come from the world of traditional Western medicine. For the past 18 years, it has been her job to help keep people free of pain, during and after surgery. But when it came to her own debilitating pain after an injury, conventional medicine was unable to help.

It happened three years ago at the end of a gallbladder operation at Union Hospital in Lynn, Massachusetts. Susan was bending over the patient's head, attempting to calm him as he began to wake up and thrash around. Somehow, his arm slipped free of the restraints, and he punched Susan so hard that she suffered a severe whiplash.

"I grabbed my neck and said, 'I've been injured,'" she recalls. "Right away my body knew that something really bad had happened."

Within days, her pain was so great that she was unable to care for herself. "I couldn't eat, I couldn't sleep, I couldn't function. My mother-in-law would come over to make dinner and help with the children and not be able to go home again for days at a time." Before long, the woman who once began her day at 4:30 a.m. with a six-mile run was spending 20 hours a day in bed, completely incapacitated.

"It was awful. My orthopedic surgeon put me on Valium and Demerol, and that took the edge off the pain for a few hours, but I had to keep on taking it for it to do any good. I knew I didn't want to become a drug addict, so I was desperate. I tried massage. I tried physical therapy. I had myself put in traction, because the only time I was comfortable was when my head was literally lifted off my body. I lost 15 pounds, I had dark circles under my eyes, my skin was gray—I didn't even look like the same person."

Finally, six grueling weeks after the accident, someone recommended acupuncture. "I said, 'I'll try anything.' So I went, and after the very first treatment, I began to feel better. I had an area of muscle spasms—literally, hard lumps that you could feel—going down my neck and back that were four inches long and about three inches wide. After the first time, those lumps became softer and softer until finally they went away."

After six weeks of acupuncture treatments, Susan's neck had healed enough to enable her to return to work. Now, three years after the accident, she has her busy, active life back. On winter weekends, Susan can be found skiing the expert trails at her favorite mountain in New Hampshire.

"I was so impressed with how I healed that now I recommend acupuncture to my own patients. My orthopedic surgeon was so amazed, he put my acupuncturist's card in his office," she says. "We need a place in medicine for this. Not everything has to be black and white. Not everything has to have 4,000 studies behind it to know that it works. *This* is the future of medicine—using the best from both worlds."

breath. If people do this five, ten minutes a day, and if they can use their diaphragmatic breathing as a way of combating stress, they enhance more pulsation in the heart. The problem with most people is this: if you're under stress, you shut off breathing. It happens all the time. If someone cuts you off on the highway, you're breathing in short shallow bursts. You do that 50, 60, 100 times a day, and you're interrupting the natural ebb and flow of pulsation, and it's pulsation which prevents disease. When we become contracted, this enhances disease.

HARRIS: So, basically you're saying the human body was designed to be open, that we should be breathing through our entire body all the time?

SINATRA: Yes. Reach out to the world. [Austrian psychiatrist] Wilhelm Reich used to say that when you reach out to the world with an open heart and open breathing, you'll prevent disease. When you become contracted, when you become fearful of the world, when you become vigilant, it's a very bad emotion because it makes us produce cortisol [a stress hormone], which causes premature aging, Alzheimer's, and other problems. That's why bioenergetics is the best-kept secret in psychotherapy, because bioenergetics opens your body up. When you open yourself up, when you open your heart, the healing is incredible. If I have a patient who falls in love at the time of an illness, whether it's cancer or heart disease or arthritis, the most healing modality you can have is the feeling of being in love. Your body vibrates with that feeling. And when that happens, your cells become healthy.

HARRIS: I want to get back for just a moment to some of the controversy about integrative medicine. What would be your response to colleagues who might say, 'I'm supposed to be working with the body. What do you mean, I have to work with the mind, too?'

SINATRA: Well, there's more and more literature written about why both are important. In fact, in 1982 we were the first to write up a paper to show that if men don't cry, they can get heart disease. We were running workshops on stress and illness; we had 40 people in the workshop and it was amazing. We were collecting urines from these people. And the women who cried in the workshop, who reached out, hugged other women and networked, had very small amounts of stress hormones in their urine. Men who built walls around themselves, didn't emote, didn't get angry, sat like stuffed shirts in a chair, didn't cry, had very high levels of stress hormones in their urine. Later we found out that these men all had heart disease. I'm convinced that the more doctors get involved with this, the more they're going to see that there is a definite mind/body connection that we should pay attention to. As a cardiologist, I call it the heart-brain hotline.

HARRIS: You say that living in awareness of your body is the key to good health. But how do you get your patients to do that?

SINATRA: That can be a tough one. This is what I tell my patients: the body always tells the truth. Most people live in denial. For example, most women think they're going to die of breast cancer, but six times as many women die of heart disease than breast cancer. That's living in denial. The same is true with the body. Whatever one thinks will affect how one feels. The problem is, many times we shut our feelings off. Every illness has a psychological and a physical component. But patients need to understand that trying to live in the brain is not healing. The healing comes when we get into the body, when we experience our body, and that's why a good doctor will integrate mind/body research to get the person into a whole aspect of healing.

HARRIS: What do you think our bodies are telling us when we get heart disease, when we get breast cancer, when we get any other disease?

SINATRA: Our bodies are telling us this: if we have heart disease, is it heartbreak? Is it being emotionally stressed out? Are we living a life full of panic? Are we living a life that's a lie? A lot of us have double lives. Their life is a lie, and they get heart disease because they're betraying their heart. What's cancer? Wilhelm Reich said that sometimes people will resign themselves to cancer as a way of getting out of life gracefully. A lot of people—not all people, now, but a lot of people—are depressed; they may unconsciously have a death wish. [Doctor] Bernie Siegel will first tell the cancer patient to fight back. You know, get into your body, use your passion, use your emotions to fight back and when these people do this, the chances of surviving cancer are better. Being a good doctor is like being a good coach. A good doctor can take a patient to a higher level, just like a good coach can take an athlete to a higher level.

HARRIS: But first the doctor has to appreciate that his or her role is, in part, to stimulate the patient's own desire to heal.

SINATRA: When a doctor or health professional nurtures a patient's own healing process, that's when miracles happen. People are powerful. We're all powerful. The body wants to be taken care of. And, remember, the body tells the truth. When you're having an illness, you've got to look at it and say, 'What did I do to influence that or create that?'

HARRIS: You'd probably get an argument on that idea, though, because some people are resistant to the idea that they have that much control over their body. That implies a tremendous amount of responsibility they may be reluctant to take.

SINATRA: And a tremendous amount of guilt. Not every person is going to create an illness. But being trained in psychotherapy and doing a lot with mind/body medicine, I can point out to a patient, about 90 to 95 percent of the time, that their emotional life, their spiritual life, their environment has really contributed to the illness. You can't force that on a patient; a patient has to be able to get that themselves. But if they get it, then the real healing will take place.

Also, it can go both ways. If I have a patient that taps into my energy, we can both have this feeling of wonderment. But sometimes you get patients who are victims, who come in and drain your energy. They will absolutely drain every ounce of vitality you have. That's when it gets to be very difficult. Many times, I'll point out to a patient that I feel like they're draining me, that I'm exhausted. That's why I have dogs in my office. If I feel drained by a patient, I'll go back

C
O
A
C
H

"Being a good doctor is like being a good coach. A good doctor can take a patient to a higher level, just like a good coach can take an athlete to a higher level."

to my little dog. I'll sit with her, make eye contact and pet her, breathe with her, and then I'm charged for the next patient. That's tapping into an animal's energy. And that, in itself, is phenomenal.

HARRIS: When you look down the road at health care, let's say 50 years from now, how different will it be then?

SINATRA: It's going to be very different. I think we're going to be seeing more naturopaths, more people who are well versed in a whole multitude of healing techniques. When a person goes to a health practitioner in the future, they're going to find a man or a woman who will sit down and talk to them, talk about their diet, talk about their stress, maybe even talk about their religious beliefs, certainly talk about their sex life and their emotional life. I'm excited about the doctors of the future, because instead of being very mechanical and having a database that's sky-high, they're going to be more grounded, in order to work on the whole patient with a holistic approach.

HARRIS: You have a son who wants to be a doctor. But you say you would recommend that he become a naturopath instead of an M.D. Why?

SINATRA: Because I think the paradigm shift in the next 10 years is going to go more towards complementary and alternative medicine. I would love it if my son became a naturopath. If you take a naturopathic doctor who has studied plants and botany, and metabolic and nutritional and emotional healing, and then put that person into a conventional medical system for a year of internship—what a powerful individual they will be. People are screaming for a health practitioner who will see them—not just their heart or their cancer or their arthritis, but see *them*. That's what people really want. The health practitioner of the future will have to sit down with the patient and see the whole patient: in their emotional, psychological, even spiritual struggle. When they do, that's when the real healing will take place.

FUTURE

"When a person goes to a health practioner in the future, they're going to find a man or a woman who will sit down and talk to them, talk about their diet, talk about their stress, maybe even talk about their religious beliefs, certainly talk about their sex life and their emotional life."

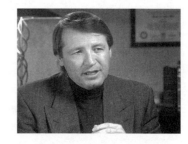

11 HEALTH AND HUNCHES: UNLOCKING YOUR INTUITION

I began using my intuition long before I knew that's what it was or had a clue about how it worked. No matter what was going on in my life, something deep within would always give me a nudge when it was time for a change: in my job, in relationships, or where I was living. Even now, when situations seem ambiguous or making a decision proves difficult, I have learned to wait until the "right" answer reveals itself. It always has—although not always as quickly as I might have preferred.

Sometimes, external events have teamed up with intuition to push me where I needed to go. When I was 25 years old, I got a job offer out of the blue to come and work for WBZ-TV in Boston. I didn't know a soul in the city and had never lived north of North Carolina. It's true, I had been feeling for the previous year that something momentous was about to happen in my life, but then I was promoted to co-anchor of the 6 p.m. news at WBTV in Charlotte, the station where I had worked for the past four years. I thought that perhaps that's what I had been feeling. Moreover, I had my eye on a house that I wanted to buy across town. Anticipating that move, I had put my little starter house on the market, but the listing with a local realtor expired with nary a nibble. No one had been interested enough to even come look at it.

Two nights after I returned to Charlotte from the job interview in Boston, not at all convinced about the wisdom of leaving the comfortable place I had carved out for myself, there came a knock at the door. A man was standing on the front steps, inquiring about the "For Sale" sign that I had neglected to remove from the front lawn. "Is your house for sale, ma'am?" he inquired. "If so, I believe I might have a buyer for you." "Uh, uh...," I stammered, not sure what to make of this amazing coincidence. "I guess it is," I finally acknowledged. A few weeks later, we had closed the deal and I was on my way north.

Years later, as I was finishing up graduate school and was in the midst of negotiating a new, three-year contract at WBZ, I found myself doing a live remote broadcast for the 5:30 news program I was co-anchoring. A celebrity chef was the featured guest that day. I had been increasingly dissatisfied with the "lite news" segments I was being asked to do, and that evening, something snapped.

"Here I am," I thought, growing more upset by the minute as I watched the fellow concocting an elaborate beef dish, "having spent thousands of dollars and hundreds of hours studying public policy—and this is how I'm supposed to use it, doing cooking segments? I don't think so." As soon as the program was over, I called my agent and told him to stop negotiating. It was time to do something else.

The decision could hardly have been scarier. I had just spent all my savings on tuition, and WBZ—which had been my professional home for five and a half years—offered a financially comfortable future. My gut, however, was screaming at me that I had to go, that I absolutely *could not* stay where I was. And even though the networks weren't hiring at the time, and my previous employment contract kept me from working anywhere else on television in Boston for nearly a year, my gut was right. After long months of unemployment, my next job turned out to be at WGBH-TV, Boston's fine public television station. For more than four years, it was the happiest and most fulfilling professional experience of my life, at least until now.

What would have happened had I not listened to my intuition, the feeling deep inside that insisted it was time to move on? Looking back, I do wonder sometimes. But after meeting physician and medical intuitive Mona Lisa Schulz—as you will, too, in this chapter—there's not much to wonder about. One way or the other, I suspect, my body would have let me know.

MONA LISA SCHULZ

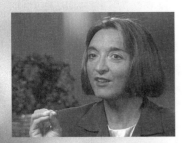

Mona Lisa Schulz, M.D., Ph.D., is a neuroscientist and physician who has also worked as a medical intuitive doing telephone consultations for more than 10 years. In addition to her medical practice, she conducts workshops for other health professionals, to help them develop their own intuitive abilities. Schulz is the author of *Awakening Intuition: Using your Mind-Body Network for Insight and Healing.*

HARRIS: Maybe we should start by trying to define what we're talking about. What, exactly, is intuition?

SCHULZ: Intuition is a sense all of us have. It's a capacity to make a correct decision with insufficient rational information. Science shows that if you have a right brain and a left brain and a body, and you sleep and dream at night, by definition you're intuitive. We've got a lot of equipment there; I've looked. All of us have the equipment to be intuitive.

HARRIS: How did you discover your intuitive abilities?

SCHULZ: I discovered them pretty much the way most people do. That is, we start in our life with a set idea, a left-brain focused idea, of who we think we are and where we think we are going. For me, it was the pursuit of intellect, because I worship at the altar of intellect, so I always thought since the age of seven that I would be in Boston and be a scientist and physician. I spent most of my adolescent and adult years trying to acquire just that. But sometimes something will happen in our health to force us to reevaluate who we think we are and where we're going. For me, my intellect stopped becoming available. I developed a sleep problem where I would walk around and fall asleep; I'd ride a bike and fall asleep in the middle of the road. I was sleeping as much as 17 and 18 hours a day while I was a student at Brown University trying to acquire my intellect. So, literally, I was spending tens of thousands of dollars in pursuit of my intellect, and I ended up having to use my intuition during those years to piece together and make sense of where I was going in my life.

What I wound up doing to heal that illness is that I began to notice when it got worse and when it got better. Naturally, I was under the care of a physician at that time, and she said, 'To some degree, Mona Lisa, even though you have a physical problem, your illness gets worse in certain situations and better in others.'

So I learned to stay awake, and I learned that my sleep attacks got worse in bad relationships when I didn't express my emotions, and got better when I stayed in good relationships. Then I went to medical school and got my M.D. and my Ph.D., and I just canned intuition. I thought, 'I am going to be a physician and scientist in a white coat with a stethoscope, working on test tubes in a lab, chopping brains for a living.' Once again, I had an idea of where I thought I was going and who I was going to be. I thought I was going to be a behavioral neurologist in a very academic environment. As far as I was concerned, you don't talk about intuition in an academic environment. You just talk about intellect. Later, when I was in Maine, my brain wanted to go into a double residency program and my body wanted to stay in Maine, and what snapped in between was my neck. So ultimately, our body in its intuition wins. We can't be driven by our head. Intuition balanced with intellect, and body balanced with brain, eventually gets harmony.

That's true for all of us. With the people I see, their body will tell them when they're in a place that needs to be evaluated, if they're in a bad relationship or a bad job, because it will act out in a certain organ system through an illness. Through ulcers or heart problems or ob/gyn problems, it will let you know through symptoms when you are going in the right direction and when you are going in the wrong direction.

H A R M O N Y

"Ultimately, our body in its intuition wins. We can't be driven by our head. Intuition balanced with intellect, and body balanced with brain, eventually gets harmony."

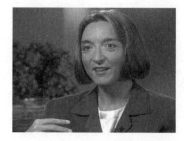

HARRIS: Why is it that women are thought to be more intuitive than men?

SCHULZ: That's a perceptual deal. That's the advertising. It's true that women are wired for cyclical intuition. Think of the right brain as the more intuitive part and the left brain as the more intellectual, rational part. Women in the first part of their cycle are mostly in their left brain, in the intellectual, rational world. Once you hit ovulation, you go more into your right brain, so women are more intuitive in their premenstrual time. That's why some people call it premenstrual syndrome, because nobody wants to hear the information that comes out then. But the problem is, that's cyclical intuition. It goes up and down. Men, however, are either in their left brain or their right brain, depending on the activity, and so men process their intuition differently. They process it in their work, and they just don't talk about it. A man might be a stock intuitive or an NBA intuitive or an athletic intuitive, able to throw the ball behind them and know who's behind them without looking. So men and women process intuition differently; one is not more intuitive than the other.

HARRIS: But as you point out in your work, their brains are organized differently.

SCHULZ: For most traditional men, their brains are compartmentalized. When they're in their left brain, they're in their left brain. When they're in their right brain, they're in their right brain. The departments in their brains are more segregated. Women go all over the brain to do tasks. They're less compartmentalized. So that's the way that I explain it. And there's a blur in between. There are definitely non-traditional men who like floral design and ballet, and their brains are slightly like women's in organization. And there are some non-traditional women, like engineers, whose brain structures are more like men's and so on. But for most women and most men, the way they approach something is different. As a result, the way they approach intuition will be different as well.

MEN/WOMEN

"Men and women process intuition differently; one is not more intuitive than the other."

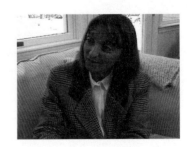

Women's brains are more like a general store, where you might be in the mop department and trip over some underwear because things are not as well compartmentalized. Men are going to be more like a department store, where the socks are going to be in a very different place from the vacuum cleaners.

HARRIS: As a scientist who has studied how the brain works, do you have any idea where intuition comes from? Is there a point in the body or in the brain that you can say, 'Aha, that's the spot?'

SCHULZ: Most of the literature suggests that some people are body intuitive. They feel it in their gut. Like I'm sure someone in the audience has a grandmother who says, 'I knew in my bones you were going to fail that exam. I told you but you didn't listen to me.' Another person will say, 'I felt it in my gut. I knew those stocks were going to go belly up, which is why I encouraged you people to sell ahead of time,' and so on. You can feel it in your chest. You can get visions. Some women got visions the day that their husband died at war. They kind of knew. Mothers know what's going on in their kid's bodies. The brain is very interesting. A study at the University of Iowa showed that a certain area in the brain, in the limbic system, is exquisitely important for intuition, and that intuition is an important sense to make reasonable, balanced decisions. When most people approach the word intuition, they think of some unusual, peculiar power. It really isn't. Intuition is something normal. It's a normal physiological process that's not just in our brain but in our body and in our sleep at night.

HARRIS: Why is it valuable?

SCHULZ: When you're born in this world, you have several senses. Wouldn't you want to use all of them? You wouldn't want to leave one behind because that would give you a direct disadvantage. So if you don't use your intuition, you're

NORMAL

"When most people approach the word intuition, they think of some unusual, peculiar power. It really isn't. Intuition is something normal."

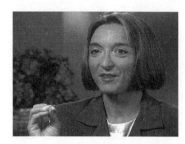

actually at a disadvantage from people who do. You're disadvantaged to make correct decisions, and you're actually disadvantaged to see potential opportunities in your life. Nurses who are experts, the thing that gives them the cutting edge over their contemporaries, is that they use intuition balanced with intellect in their clinical duties to make better decisions. In fact, those nurses try to teach this to the beginning nurses. Doctors use it. It gives them that extra hunch. It gives them the sense of where they need to go the extra mile for a patient. In ancient Greece, intuition and dreams used to be a part of the medical school, which is really an interesting thing. I guess they kind of worked it out of the curriculum. But I hope that someday soon, physicians in medical schools, people in MBA programs—in almost every profession—will learn to use intuition with their other senses to make balanced clinical or career decisions.

When I was first in the hospital, I figured I'd leave intuition at home. I wanted to be Joe Professional. I got the white coat, the starch, the new stethoscope, the ophthalmoscope, I don't even know how to use it. I shine the light in my own eyes and it almost blinds me. So this is not inspiring confidence in my patients. But I do have what we call auxiliary frontal lobes, auxiliary intellect. So I would look around the hospital, and I would know that there were some nurses who always knew what was going to happen, especially when you sign up to be on call at four o'clock. There was always one nurse, I'd go up to her and say, 'So what's going to happen tonight?' And she'd say, 'Oh, tonight's going to be okay.' And you could just relax and get books to read. Other nights she'd say, 'Better stay close by Mary Brown, down the hallway.' And I'd say, 'Is it her vital signs?' Because I'm looking for data. She'd say, 'No.' 'Is it her skin color?' 'Nope.' 'EKG?' 'Nope.' 'Chest x-ray?' 'Uh-uh.' 'What is it?' She says, 'I just know.' And unerringly, seven o'clock, code red on the lady.

In the intensive care unit, I would sit there and I would watch all these beeps go off, because everyone is wired with all these warning bells. You can roll over and the warning bell goes off. You think an evil thought, the warning bell goes off. Whatever happens to the patient, the warning bell goes off. These nurses would never get up. They learn how to conserve their energy, and they learn how to know what buzzer was real and what buzzer was artificial. At around four o'clock they would be sitting around the table with the pork-fried rice and the chicken wings, and they would be sitting there eating them casually. The buzzers would go off and I would exhaust myself, because I would run for every buzzer. They would just sit there and eat their food. And then one buzzer

Christiane Northrup

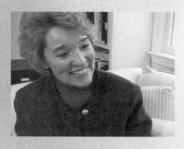

Christiane Northrup, M.D., founder of the innovative healthcare center, Women to Women in Yarmouth, Maine, has been working side by side with Mona Lisa Schulz for the past six years. She is herself a well-known figure in the field of emotions and health, who both believes in and welcomes the use of intuition in medical practice.

"I believe that all of us are intuitive," says Dr. Northrup. "We don't pay any attention to it because our society doesn't validate it. But all good doctors use it, and in fact, all humans use it. It's just that it isn't 'named,' and naming has great power."

During a consultation with a new patient, Dr. Northrup first asks, "What do *you* think is going on?" Then, if the patient seems open to the idea, "I bring in what they need to do to access their inner wisdom, their intuition." Often she will recommend an invitation to self-discovery, in much the same way that she would prescribe medicine.

"A prescription is the symbol of the Western medical interaction. You hand your patient a prescription for a medication: 'Our time is up, Mrs. Jones, you now have your Valium....' What I do by writing down, 'Do a meditation on nurturance,' for example, means that I am not ending my consultation with, 'This is the drug that will save you,' I'm ending with, 'This is how you're going to make a contribution to your own healing.' There may well be a drug that's helpful for this condition, and that's fine; that's the bridge they walk across. What I do is stimulate their own knowing about what caused their illness by validating it in a Western way, with a stethoscope around my neck. It gives patients permission to explore what they already know."

Dr. Northrup continues to marvel at how her colleague is able to add another dimension to medical practice by using her intuitive abilities. "Time and time again, we go to the operating room and what Mona Lisa has 'seen,' as it were, we then see in surgery, or I see on a blood test. So I don't need to be convinced that she has a gift. If I'm in Europe, she can sense what's going on with me. This is not a gift I have. Or, actually, I believe that I have it but it's not developed yet, for whatever reason."

What originally sparked Dr. Northrup's interest in listening to the body's inner voice was an illness of her own. As a physician, wife, and mother of two, her schedule kept her going at a dizzying pace. "I was exhausted, my face was all broken out, and then I developed a breast

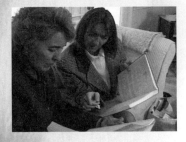 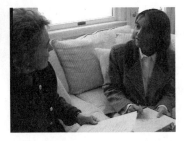 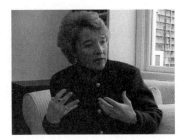

abscess which pretty much ruined the function of my right breast. I knew enough about mind/body interaction to know that the breast abscess was related to germs, and also related to my own inner wisdom trying to tell me something about taking care of myself."

In fact, observes Dr. Northrup, "It is usually illness, or something that is very painful, that gets us to wake up. What I'm doing now in my life is trying to teach people to make this change *before* a major illness or a major accident. Whether you change things sooner or later, your life is not whole until you do."

would go off among the symphony of bells, and they'd all drop their chicken wings and go running. And I would say, 'How did you know that? How do you know what buzzers are real and which ones aren't?' And they'd say, 'We just know.' They were the ones that were seasoned; they were the expert nurses. They were the ones that were a cut above the others.

HARRIS: When you do a consultation as a medical intuitive, how does that work? I mean, if you're speaking to someone who you think has a heart problem, do you feel a heaviness in your chest?

SCHULZ: I have two jobs. One is that I'm a physician, very traditional. They come in, they get diagnosed, they get treated, they get their medicines. The other job is working with people who don't want a physician. In fact, they sign a release form that acknowledges I'm not doing that. I'm not diagnosing or treating them. What they want is someone who knows only their name and their age and doesn't see them, to educate them on what specific situations are going on in their emotional life, what specific situations are going on in certain organs of their body. Given someone's name and their age, I can, in my mind's eye, see specific situations that are going on in their emotional life, be it a situation with their relationship, a specific situation at work and so on. And then I can see it through the body, their head, heart, left breast, right breast, GI tract, pelvic, and in their skeletal system. I can see in what area they're experiencing symptoms, I can describe the symptoms, and then I can relate what specific symptoms are going on in their physical body with what's going on in their emotional life. At the end I say, 'Does this make sense?' Because I'm balancing, now, my intellect with my intuition. And they say, for example, 'Yes, I knew that nameless discomfort in my abdomen was telling me for years that something was wrong with my job, and I refused to listen to it. I refused to watch that warning light on my dashboard of life. And as a result, this went on for years, and I eventually developed an ulcer.' Then I describe to them the scientific studies that are associated with that particular case, like ulcers and a competitive spirit at work. And then this person says, 'Oh my God, what I thought was going on in my body—there's actually science to support that?' And I say, 'Yes, and it shows that people who learn to change how they approach their work and try to smooth over their competitive spirit, their ulcers can get better.'

HARRIS: Were you surprised when you first began being able to make these connections?

SCHULZ: Yes, I was. I was at Boston City Hospital. I was a medical student, and I had just finished most of my M.D. and most of my Ph.D., and I was there to start working on patients as they came into the emergency room. What's now known as Boston Medical Center used to be Boston City Hospital. And I think you know the way it used to be; it was unbelievable. People would throw patients at you and say, 'Mary Brown, 48, she's in the emergency room, pick her up, she's yours,' and they were out of there. There was not enough information. There was never enough information, and no one had time to give you enough information. So on my way down to the ER in my white coat I would say, 'Okay, Mary Brown, 48,' and then I would just get this image in my mind. I would think probably she's moderately obese, she's got green stretch pants. I would see Mary Brown. And I would say, 'Oh. She thinks it's gallbladder.' So on the way down to the ER—the elevators were really slow and congested at that time—I would get agitated, so I did this little exercise on my clipboard. I'd say, 'Okay, what would I do if someone had gallbladder problems? I'll need to get her to radiology, get her an ultrasound, check the whites of her eyes to see if she's jaundiced.' So I would write this down on my clipboard. By the time I got to the ER, I'd pull the curtain over her, and there she was, Mary Brown, lying on the gurney with these green stretch pants, clutching the right side of her upper abdomen, saying, 'Doctor, doctor, it's my gallbladder.' What was odd was that I did this several days in a row. And I used to get out earlier than all the other people, because it was like a shortcut. I would know ahead of time what would be wrong with my patients, and it would help me work them up faster. All the other medical students got angry because they said, 'How do you get out so fast?' What I learned was that the best people there were the ones who were the most knowledgeable and made the best decisions, because they were also using their intuition.

When I work as an intuitive now, I try to immediately teach people how to listen to their intuition and their own body. That is, I'm teaching them to wake up to the signals in their body that are telling them through illness that something in their life needs to change. Most people say, 'Yeah, I got a sense of that,' but they turn that speaker down. They'd rather go with the idea that, 'I'm going to keep this job because it makes me a lot of money, and it makes me feel powerful in the world.' They are going to turn the speaker down of that nameless discomfort in their body that's edging them toward the idea that maybe there's another job they should be doing, one that's more in keeping with health.

HARRIS: What does that tell you about the diseases we acquire?

SCHULZ: Well, here's what happened to me. I spent my whole life trying to learn how the intellect works. I ended up, as a result, learning how to treat patients with problems with their brain. Eventually I stumbled upon the fact that there are additional ways of accessing one's mind, one's intellect. One of those is intuition. But it came to me through the study and healing of my own brain. Another scientist might work to understand the illnesses that his mother suffers and so on. We are driven to study and heal the very things in our life that give us pain and suffering at first, but then bring us healing.

I tried to go into neurology, because I thought that was it. I thought all the mind was in neurology because they literally had the brains in the lab, and I

S I G N A L S

"When I work as an intuitive now, I try to immediately teach people how to listen to their intuition and their own body... to wake up to the signals in their body that are telling them through illness that something in their life needs to change."

wanted to be intelligent. First time I tried to go into neurology, I pulled two disks in my neck and got paralysis in my hand. I waited two years to go into psychology, then I decided to go into neurology again and blew two more disks. Four disks, multiple hospital bills—what do you think? My dreams were telling me to reevaluate how I looked at myself, and my body was telling me, too. I go away from a career that my brain thought I wanted to be in, my body gets better. I go toward the career that my brain thought I was going to be in, my body gets worse. Clearly, if I don't look at this compass, I could be losing more disks down the road, and I don't have that many left. The point is, we have to listen to our bodies. Men in certain jobs, when they grow old they start to get heart problems. Women, in relationships that are not nurturing, tend to be at a higher risk for breast cancer. The next question that people ask is, 'OK, so does that mean that I caused my disk to blow?' And, 'Did I cause my breast cancer?' The answer is no, because emotions in our brain release chemicals, the same chemicals that organs in our body produce when they function. Emotion occurs in the brain, and it occurs at the same time in the body with symptoms. So the reality is, if an emotion or a situation in our life is unhealed, our body at the same time will act up. Our symptoms tell us it needs to be healed. We are not to blame for our illnesses, but we are able to be responsive to them. They are like a compass pointing us in the direction for health.

HARRIS: So this is important information our bodies are giving us. They're saying, 'Yes, you really do want to do this,' or 'No, maybe not.'

SCHULZ: Here's another example. Men who have had a heart attack, that disease has been associated with problems with emotional expression, of getting stuck on one channel or flavor of emotion: hostility. Believe it or not, they have an instrument to measure hostility; I don't know how they do it, but they do it. Anyway, these men who have had a heart attack are put in groups to teach them other ways of expressing themselves, so they can release their hostility.

C O M P A S S

"We are not to blame for our illnesses, but we are able to be responsive to them. They are like a compass pointing us in the direction for health."

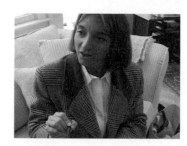

Ann-Marie Almeida

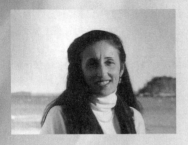

L I F E

It took nine months and a number of cancelled appointments before Ann-Marie Almeida finally connected with Dr. Mona Lisa Schulz for an intuitive reading over the telephone.

"I didn't really believe in it, so I kept kind of putting it off. But I was curious. Eventually, I decided to give it a try," recalls Ann-Marie, who had been diagnosed with a large fibroid tumor next to her uterus three years previously. "When we spoke on the phone, I gave her my name and age. That was all.

"Dr. Schulz started at the top of my head and at first she said, 'Why are you calling, you look like a healthy person.' Then she got to my abdomen and she said, 'Oh. I can see a dark fibrous mass, and it's starting to affect your kidneys, colon, and digestive tract'—which was exactly what my doctor had told me."

Ann-Marie's doctor had also advised her to have the tumor removed, but Ann-Marie was reluctant. She had been diagnosed with a smaller tumor in 1992, and it had gone away on its own. Ann-Marie, a Reiki Master with years of healing experience, believed it was possible to make this tumor disappear, too. She was at least determined to try.

Dr. Schulz told her otherwise. "She was so clear," says Ann-Marie. "She said, 'No, you can't cure it yourself. You've got to have it out.'"

A few months later, Ann-Marie did. The eight-pound fibroid tumor was removed in July of 1998, one day before she turned 40.

But Ann-Marie got more than medical advice from Dr. Schulz. "She said I needed to clean up my emotional act and reclaim my life as a powerful woman who makes good decisions. She also said my dissatisfaction with my job was making the situation worse and that I should quit, which I did.

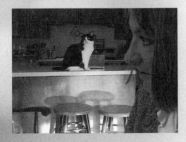
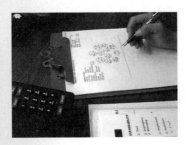
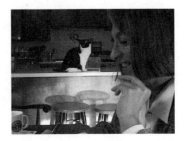

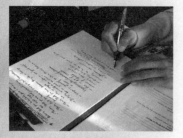

"What struck me most about Mona Lisa was her integrity. She didn't mince words; she was painfully honest. It's clear that her mission is to help people by giving them some important information. At the end, I was in tears because she had described me so accurately. She gave me a new way of understanding myself, especially my emotional life, that I hadn't had before. Just before we hung up, I asked her what I should do. She said, 'Do what you want.' She obviously sees it as her job to tell you what you need to know, and then it's up to you whether you do anything about it or not."

Seven months after her operation, Ann-Marie reports, she's back in good health, with a new job she enjoys, and a different perspective on her life.

"I wanted so much to heal myself that I had totally lost sight of the fact that it didn't have to be either/or. As it turned out, the surgery was an important part of my beginning to heal my life in other ways."

Those men actually live longer and have fewer heart attacks than the ones who continue on their merry way having problems with hostility. So there are life-saving and life-healing reasons why one would want to listen to intuition and how your body speaks to you.

HARRIS: Are children naturally more intuitive than adults?

SCHULZ: The area in our brain that's important for intuition is the area in the temporal lobe and a small area above it. This area develops in all of us when we are very young. However, there's an area in the frontal lobe that doesn't come on board until later on in life, after puberty. So, as children, we have more access to our intuition, because the area in our frontal lobe that doubts our intuition is not on board yet. Think of it as your frontal lobe that says, 'You can't possibly know this, you can't do this, you're foolish.' The inner critic is always talking inside of us and balancing the other part of the brain that says, 'Don't you get a sense that relationship or that job is wrong for you?' And so we have to balance the temporal-lobe intuition with the frontal-lobe inner critic to make correct decisions. But children don't have enough frontal lobe yet, so they don't have that inner Judge Judy that says, 'You can't know this, it's not right, it's not the rules.' They have what we call unbridled intuition.

As adults, the problem is that we fall in line, we want to be socially appropriate, we want to get our pay raises and we don't want the IRS after us. So we do what we think we ought to do, rather than what our body senses. As a result, as we get older, sometimes intuition is harder to access.

HARRIS: So if a child says something that seems very intuitive, should the parent encourage them?

SCHULZ: Well, here's the issue. Some kids who have ADD [attention deficit disorder], who are hyperactive and impulsive, actually the frontal-lobe programs for inhibiting socially inappropriate behavior are not there real well. Kids who have hyperactivity and ADD tend to be impulsive and blurt out their intuitive perceptions. So one kid, the father comes home on a Friday night, and the kid says, 'Daddy, that perfume smells so good, how come you won't get Mommy perfume like that?' And the father's, like, kicking the kid. And the mother says, 'John, perfume?' And the kid says, 'No, no, it's wonderful, Mommy. You should have Daddy buy you that perfume.' Kids will blurt things out, especially kids with hyperactivity and ADD. Adults, too, will blurt out intuition. But it will appear at times to be socially inappropriate and make other people uncomfortable.

HARRIS: If someone wanted to tap into her own intuitive abilities, is it hard? Does it take a long time? How do you do it?

SCHULZ: Tapping into it is a good way to put it. Adjusting the reception and turning up the volume is another way of saying it. Think of intuition as another sense you have. It's like a radio transmitter in your back pocket that at any time is broadcasting information. What you simply need to do is turn up the volume and adjust your reception of intuition. The way to do that is to find out what area of your brain, your body, or in sleep that you process intuition. If you're a right-handed, left-brain dominant person, that means you love reading, you love writing. Chances are you are a left-brain intuitive, and that means your intuition will come primarily to you through dreams that are symbolic. In fact, the literature suggests that certain dreams can tell you ahead of time what's going to happen in your body. Some women have had dreams of little rats taking nips out of their stomach. Two months later, they get an ulcer. So: left-brain intuitives, if you write a lot, love symbolic language, love poetry, love the analogy of writing and reading, then chances are you could turn up the volume through dreams. However, maybe you are not that way. Maybe you're like me.

Developing Intuition

Want to develop your own intuitive powers? Psychotherapist and intuitive Belleruth Naparstek, author of *Your Sixth Sense: Unlocking the Power of Your Intuition*, recommends the following practices:

1   **Meditate regularly** to clear and still your mind and to focus your awareness. Lovingkindness (metta) meditation and heart-opening guided imagery are especially powerful and trustworthy ways to expand intuitive ability.

2   **Exercise regularly** to ensure a fit body for handling the increased energy that moves through your system when you do intuitive work.

3   **Create sacred space.** Either set aside a special area of your home or office in which to practice intuition exercises, or establish a ritual surrounding your time of seeking intuitive guidance.

4   **Set your intention** on opening to intuition in a trustworthy, respectful way that is focused on service, not power.

5   **Test your intuitive ability** on things that don't matter, like predicting which bank teller will open up next, or who's calling on the phone. When there's no pressure to perform, abilities open up.

6   **Keep track of how your body feels** when you get an accurate intuitive hit. How does that differ from the feeling of a "miss"?

7   **Keep a journal** of intuitive experiences, recording your daily hits and misses. You'll start to see patterns, what time of day or month your intuition is enhanced; how diet, emotions, geographic location—even the company you keep—affect your intuitive abilities.

8   **Verify your experiences** with objective data. This will help you avoid distorting information received intuitively.

9   **Know yourself.** Self-awareness helps you separate intuition from projections of your own wishes and fears. Mindfulness meditation, psychotherapy, or regular introspection with a friend, support group, or teacher can help eliminate blocks, self-deception, and distractions that prevent you from receiving clear, direct information. Still, don't assume you'll be right all the time; no one is.

10   **Tell the truth.** Intuitive awareness is about integrity—being true to your inner experience. The more truthful you are with yourself and others, the less you will be at the mercy of outside influences, and the more you will be able to rely on your intuitive abilities.

11   **Slow down and seek out solitude.** Quiet time alone allows for greater intuition and helps you rebalance and stay grounded.

12   **Work continually on opening your heart.** Practice kindness and forgiveness. You'll not only become more intuitive, but you'll be a trustworthy carrier of the information you receive.

You are probably another kind of intuitive, you may be a right-brain intuitive or a body intuitive. You will experience intuition maybe through seeing things, or hearing sounds, or sensing things in your body. So you need to find out how your body and your brain process intuition.

HARRIS: What would you say to someone who would hear of the kind of work you do as a medical intuitive and say, 'Oh, I could never do anything like that.'

SCHULZ: In 1984, right around that time, a woman named Barbara Brennen came out with a book called *Hands of Light*, where they have people lying down and they heal through the chakras, which are energy centers in the body. And she sees and she feels and she uses her hands. I look at this book and I think, 'I don't see chakras, and I'm not particularly intuitive,' and I close the book. I mean, I wouldn't know a chakra, I've never seen a chakra, I wouldn't know one if I tripped over it. The reality is, if you look at other people's particular gifts and talents you will not be able to see your own.

My intuition, I see things. Other people will feel things in their body—that's clairsentient. Some people get the most amazing dreams of solutions to experiments in the lab and so on. One famous scientist discovered the carbon atom, the benzene ring, through a dream where he saw a snake with his mouth and his tail in his hand. So the idea is not to look and focus on how another person may process intuition, but to focus on how you yourself do. The other thing is, we tend to be less able at times to see our own health issues clearly. I'm not the best intuitive for myself, which is a shame because I've had health problems, but I can see health really easily for other people. I guess you might say that I have turned down the volume and the reception on my own health, but I'm working on it. That's why sharing your intuition with others, in balance with intellect, is important. But each of us has our own unique gifts and talents.

HARRIS: There are those who believe that the next major step forward for us as a species is to be able to use our intuitive abilities as easily as we use our other five senses. What's your take on that?

SCHULZ: When I worked for my Ph.D., some of what I learned was the development of the brain, how the brain evolved over time. What some scientists believe is that the left brain is more evolved, that it's gotten bigger and bigger and that our brain has gotten more compartmentalized. A right-handed man's brain is supposed to be the most highly evolved, because the left brain is

supposed to be a lot bigger and it's supposed to have all these neat compart-
ments. In addition, we think that the brain developed along a line where more
symbolic language is important. Think of it as a web, that we've developed this
capacity in our brain to process and communicate information. I think the next
step is to then learn the proper context within which to use that information
and communicate it. And that's where the right brain comes in, because the
right brain has intense connections to the body, emotion, and spirituality.
Using that resource, funneling it over to the left brain, and using our wonderful communication skills that have developed and evolved over time to communicate this knowledge and wisdom, is, I think, the next step. Balancing
intuition from our body and our brains with the intellect that we have developed over our lifetime, is, I think, where our evolution is going.

HARRIS: You were speaking earlier about women's intuitive abilities fluctu-
ating according to their cycle. If those abilities are tied to their menstrual
cycles, what happens after menopause?

SCHULZ: Pre-ovulatory, we're in our left brain, listening to things in the
world. After ovulation, our right brain is more turned on, and we're more open
to intuition. So think of it as strobe-light intuition before menopause: off/on,
off/on. What happens at menopause is, it's no longer strobe. The light is stuck
on. It's static intuition. And so that's why it might have been in ancient soci-
eties that after a woman went through menopause she was considered a wise
woman. She was wired for the wisdom of the world. Now, men might say, what
about me, I don't have ovaries. Maybe it's the only time in their whole life they
wish they had a menstrual cycle. The reality is that men process intuition differently. At the beginning of their life, their attention and reaction in the world
is what we call impulsive; they'll see a target and they'll shoot. A woman waits
and then shoots. So a woman is more likely through the beginning of her life
to get information, wait and then act on it. At menopause and testopause—
because men go through the same kind of hormonal change in their 50s—
men's cognition becomes a little more like women's. So they're more likely to
wait, to be more receptive to intuition, and then make more accurate shots at
the goal. Our brains are wired for intuition differently throughout our lifetimes, through childhood, through the reproductive years and through
menopause and testopause.

HARRIS: It sounds as if they begin to intersect a bit in their 50s.

s c h u l z : In fact, that's what happens. Men have a more masculinized-style intuition and then it gets more feminized as they get into testopause in their 50s. The opposite is true of women. Women are born with a more feminine style of intuition, and as they get to menopause, it becomes more male-oriented. The thing is, we intersect at menopause and testopause in our 50s. So it's true. How we are as individuals, our gender identity, changes throughout our lifetime, and so does intuition.

h a r r i s : And all of us have it, even if we're not sure that's what it is?

s c h u l z : There's a woman who called me up who was doing a television show a few years ago and she said, 'You're a medical intuitive. Do a reading for me on the phone right now.' And I said, 'Isn't your program trying to show people how to use their own intuition?' She said 'Yes.' And I said, 'I could do one for you right now, but that's not the point. If I do that, it's a focus on what my brand of intuition is, and it really doesn't help you get in touch with yours.' And she said, 'Oh.' She seemed somewhat disinterested, and then we talked about other things. In the middle of the talk her voice got hoarse, and she got worse and worse. After 20 minutes she said, 'I have to get off the phone. My neck is in a tremendous amount of pain, I feel like I'm choking.' She gets off the phone, saying she'd call me the next day. And I'm thinking this is, 'Don't call me, I'll call you,' because I didn't give her what she wants, I didn't do a performance. The next day she called me up and her voice sounded completely different. She said, 'I have to tell you the most amazing thing. The moment I got on the phone with you, my neck was killing me. It got worse and worse. And when I got off the phone, it went away. Now, I've never had a problem in my neck before, but can you please tell me, do you have problems with your neck?' And I said, 'Do I have problems with my neck?!' I told her, 'Guess what. You're a medical intuitive like all of us. You have a body, you have a brain, you sleep at night, you're clairsentient, you experience things in your body—and now you have something to talk about on your show.'

All of us need to learn how we process intuition, whether we feel it in the body, which is clairsentient; or we see things, which is clairvoyant; or we dream, which is intuitive. We all have this capacity.

12 PEAK PERFORMANCE: SPORTS AND THE MIND

There are few things more satisfying to the amateur athlete than the solid *thwack* of a tennis ball as it's propelled off the sweet spot of a racket, the satisfying *swoosh* as a basketball cuts through the netting without touching the hoop, or the high arc of a cleanly hit golf ball as it flies off the tee and travels 250 yards down the fairway.

In those moments, we get a glimpse—if only for the briefest of instants—what it must feel like to be Steffi Graf, or Michael Jordan, or Greg Norman. Obviously, the vast majority of us will never know the satisfaction of being a world champion in tennis, or basketball, or golf. But there are ways that we can improve what we do at any level in sports, by using the power of our minds to enhance the performance of our bodies. In this chapter, sports psychologist George Mumford shares with us some of the winning secrets he has used with the Chicago Bulls for the past five years. The secret begins with the intention of our thoughts, as we attempt to connect to "the zone"—one of those phrases that's easy to toss off, but as any athlete can attest, difficult to achieve.

Here again, mindfulness is the key: being "fully present in the moment," as Mumford tries to be, in every aspect of his life.

It's true, mindfulness by itself is unlikely to turn the weekend warrior into a world-class athlete. But even if it only brings us greater clarity, more satisfaction, and less frustration in our own athletic pursuits, that's not such a bad deal either.

GEORGE MUMFORD

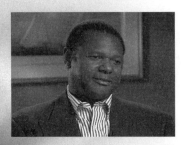

George Mumford works as a sports psychologist and organizational development consultant. For the past five years, he has been a consultant to the six-time NBA champion Chicago Bulls, working with players like Michael Jordan, Scotty Pippen and Dennis Rodman, both individually and as a team. He has also worked with the Boston College basketball team. In addition, Mumford has taught meditation and mindfulness techniques to people recovering from drug and alcohol abuse, including prison inmates in Massachusetts. The circumstances of his students may be different, says Mumford, but the message they absorb is equally important.

HARRIS: When most of us look at an athletic performance, we tend to think about it as a magnificently conditioned body doing something amazing. What does the mind have to do with it?

MUMFORD: I would say the mind has everything to do with it and very little to do with it. It's sort of a paradox. What I mean is, if the mind can just settle back and take second place and allow the body to do its thing, it's not a problem. But if the mind gets involved too much, it can impact the performance of the body doing the movements it needs to do. The mind has everything to do with it, from the standpoint of forming the intention and directing the body, and then allowing the body to do its thing without over-control.

HARRIS: Over-control. So what you're suggesting is that sometimes the mind can get in the way of what the body is trying to do.

MUMFORD: That's right.

HARRIS: How do you keep that from happening?

MUMFORD: By understanding how the mind and body work together optimally, and getting them to work in harmony instead of working against each other. A lot of that has to do with clarity of thought, as well as preparing or training the body to react under certain circumstances and certain situations, so that there isn't the need to think about what you're doing. You just react to the situation. Thinking stops the activity or the movement of the body, especially if you need to make very quick decisions, whether it's in sports or anything else in life—like when somebody cuts you off in traffic. You have to understand how to train yourself so that when that situation happens, you're able to make the right decision.

HARRIS: I want you to think back to day one, when you went in to meet with the Chicago Bulls. These players have probably never heard of you, they don't really know what you're there for. What do you say to them?

MUMFORD: I talk to them about possibilities. I talk to them about the fact that as human beings we only use a small percentage of our potential, depending on who you talk to and what literature you read. You can get anywhere from one percent to 10 percent of your brain capability, with Einstein being someone who's using 10 percent of his capacity. Looking at it from a developmental point of view, what I suggest is that no matter where you are, there's room for improvement. The more we can be in the moment, the more effective we are. One way of harnessing that untapped potential is to learn how to use the mind in conjunction with the body.

HARRIS: Specifically, how do you do that?

MUMFORD: I use role models, or I use people who seem to be operating on a more optimal level—people who seem to be creating in the moment. If you were to ask them how did they know what to do, they would say, 'I just did.' But I know from experience that they go over some of those moves in practice, in non-game situations. Then when the game situation occurs, they can actually move beyond that, if their mind status is proper, and if they're able to sense what's going on and allow the body to do its thing. I suggest that there are ways of being more effective—when mind, body, and spirit are in harmony. What I mean by spirit is energy or exuberance, that sort of thing. There are ways we relate to our experience that increase energy, and other ways that decrease energy. Also, once you have that energy, how do you control it? That's another component in terms of understanding how to regulate your emotions.

HARRIS: Good question. How do you control them?

MUMFORD: It's not that simple. It depends on the situation and the person, and it usually has to do with what we think. For instance, if you're competing and you have a thought that says, 'I can't do this,' or, 'That's too difficult for me,' those thoughts actually change the chemical makeup of your body. You can lose energy or you can get into a place where you're not able to do what you're trying to do. The opposite is also true. If you have confidence and you say, 'I'm going to do this,' and you have what I call positive self-talk, then you see that the energy increases, and you're actually able to do it. It's a mystery in terms of how it happens, but I know that there are things we do that seem to create the environment or conditions for those type of experiences to happen. There's a lot of training involved, in terms of using the mind or clearing the mind to the point that you're more effective. Arnold Schwarzenegger said once about lifting weights that if he has one lift with total consciousness, it's equal to 10 lifts when he's not totally conscious. That says a lot. There's something about the quality of mind that enhances the experience. I don't know how else to say it.

HARRIS: When it comes to mindfulness, very often it's taught through the breath. If you are very deliberate in how you take a breath, then that will help you be in the moment. Is that the kind of thing you tell these athletes to do as well?

MUMFORD: Yes. I use the breath because the breath is always present. The breath seems to be able to harmonize the mind and the body. It doesn't have to be the breath, as long as it's one thing that the mind is focused on. But the breath works perfectly, because it's what we have and it's available all the time.

HARRIS: Does it help people focus?

"If you're competing and you have a thought that says, 'I can't do this,' or, 'That's too difficult for me,' those thoughts actually change the chemical makeup of your body."

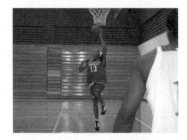

MUMFORD: If they focus on breathing in and breathing out, yes. It's something you have to train, like lifting weights. You can't just do it without training the mind to do it, so that when you're in a situation and need it, it's there.

HARRIS: What are some of the other examples you use when you're working, particularly with elite athletes who might say, 'What are you talking about, George? I'm not sure about this.'

MUMFORD: Well, what seems to work very well is having them recall a situation or a time when they seemed to be in the zone, as they say, when things were going smoothly and they were performing well. When I ask them to describe some of the qualities in that feeling, then that gives us a basis for talking about what's possible when there's more training. So instead of having it happen haphazardly, it can happen with more frequency.

HARRIS: So that they're doing it on purpose.

MUMFORD: They're doing it on purpose, right. I'm not sure how you get into the zone. I think that breathing allows you access to it. It's more efficient in terms of being able to move into the zone, because there are certain characteristics that you experience when you're in the zone. One is relaxed concentration—being in the moment and seeing things as they are without being reactive to them. But at the same time there's a sense that you're seeing what's happening and you can respond to it. Let's say you're playing basketball or tennis. It may take numerous repetitions, but then you find yourself sometimes where the racket is doing its thing by itself or the basket seems very big, where there's a harmonizing with what you're doing. You're totally in the moment. For whatever reason, everything is in rhythm, working with each other rather than at cross purposes. We don't get that experience very often, but when you do, you have a sense that there's something wondrous happening. I think as spectators when we observe athletic competition, we sometimes see that. There's a magic moment when you get to see how things just flow.

HARRIS: What about the everyday athlete, though, all of us weekend warriors. Can we do this, too?

MUMFORD: Absolutely. We have the same body. We have the same mind. The question is: how are we using our energy? Are we learning how to focus the mind? Are we doing activities to develop high skill levels, where we're creating the conditions so that every once in a while we have that experience of feeling fully alive? It doesn't have to be athletics. It can be conversation. It can be listening to a child, or doing some work. What seems to be necessary is that we develop a certain skill level of paying attention, instead of the body being here and the mind being out in the stands, you might say, if you're performing on the tennis court or basketball court or hockey rink. Or if you're at work at your computer and your mind is somewhere else. It isn't the same as when you feel your mind and your fingers being there, feeling that energy of being in the moment and really feeling connected.

HARRIS: Do you recommend meditation to the athletes you work with as a way of getting to that feeling?

MUMFORD: I do. I recommend meditation, but I don't always call it meditation. Sometimes I call it just being aware of breathing or breathing with awareness. The idea is to learn how to focus the mind, because a lot of us are meditating even though we may not know it. Whatever thoughts are dominant in your mind, you're meditating on that. If you're involved in criminal activity, or if you're a substance abuser and you're thinking about getting drugs or alcohol, that's what you focus on. That's what you're meditating on, and your behavior will demonstrate that. A lot of us are meditating on thoughts that we're not even aware of, but those thoughts are taking us places.

HARRIS: So if you want to perform well athletically, do you have to concentrate on what you want to have happen and not allow yourself to think of anything else?

MUMFORD:: Not only on what you want to have happen, but what's present in your mind. What are your thoughts? How do your thoughts affect your feelings and how do your feelings affect your behavior? That way, you learn how this mind/body process operates, by seeing what thoughts are predominant and making a conscious choice to maybe change those thoughts. If they're negative thoughts, then you're going to have negative effects or negative feelings. If

ATTENTION

"What seems to be necessary is that we develop a certain skill level of paying attention, instead of the body being here and the mind being out in the stands, you might say, if you're performing on the tennis court or basketball court or hockey rink."

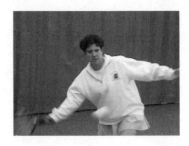

Phil Jackson

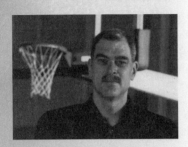

The world may know Phil Jackson as the coach who led the Chicago Bulls to six championships in eight years, but that isn't necessarily how he sees himself. Beyond all the accolades of his career, Jackson's life is focused on ideas like mindfulness, becoming a peaceful warrior, plugging into the power of oneness. Not the usual bill of fare in the intensely competitive world of professional sports.

The son of two deeply religious parents—his mother a Pentecostal evangelist, his father a pastor at a number of churches in Montana—Jackson's early life followed the rhythms of the church: services on Wednesday and Friday evenings, Sundays devoted to spiritual activities.

In his early teens, Jackson experienced a crisis of sorts with his faith. Baseball and basketball became his new passions. The summer after his freshman year in college, Jackson felt something pop in his shoulder while pitching for an American Legion team. His brother Joe, a Ph.D. candidate in psychology, guided Phil through a series of self-hypnosis and auto-suggestion exercises as part of his recuperation.

Of his return to the mound, Jackson said, "That day I discovered that I could be effective, even overcome pain, by letting go and not thinking. It was an important turning point for me." That summer, Jackson also encountered Zen Buddhism through his brother. It turned out to be a life-transforming introduction.

In 1967, Jackson got a job offer from the New York Knicks, the team where he would spend the next 11 years playing alongside the likes of Bill Bradley, Walt Frazier, and Earl Monroe. It was there that he began absorbing the philosophies of coach Red Holzman, such as: awareness is everything, don't let anger cloud the mind, the power of "we" is greater than the power of "me."

By the end of his playing days, he was well into a serious study of meditation and other spiritual practices. When he became head coach of the Chicago Bulls in 1989, he had the chance to put his off-court ideas into practice on the court. His first move was to institute the triangle offense, based on the Taoist principle of yielding to an opponent's force in order to render him powerless. "It embodied the Zen/Christian attitude of selfless awareness," recalls Jackson. "In essence, the system was a vehicle for integrating mind and body,

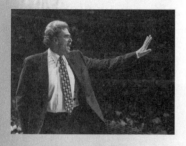

sport and spirit in a practical, down-to-earth form that anyone could learn. It was awareness in action."

His vision of total mindfulness for the Bulls went even farther. Practices were sacred places where only Bulls players and coaches were permitted. The team room was decorated with Native American totems, to celebrate the Lakota Sioux concept of teamwork. Players gathered in a circle at the beginning and end of practice as a symbol of their selfless commitment to their mission. Meditation was practiced; visualization techniques used.

The rest, as they say, is history. Six NBA titles in eight years.

"Like life, basketball is messy and unpredictable," says Jackson. "It has its way with you, no matter how hard you try to control it. The trick is to experience each moment with a clear mind and open heart. When you do that, the game—like life—will take care of itself."

they're positive thoughts, then they're going to lead to positive feelings and positive behaviors. It's not as simple as just changing your thinking; it's also looking at our belief systems or how we view the world. For instance, if you view the world as a place where things happen to you and you are just a victim, then your behavior is going to be different from someone who is proactive and feels like no matter what the world presents them, they can choose to respond in a way where they can get their needs met and get some satisfaction. So it's a very different frame of reference.

HARRIS: Sometimes before an athletic performance, you get to see a close-up of someone on television, and you will see this very intense, very focused look on the athlete's face. What's going on in there? What do you think that person is thinking?

MUMFORD: My suspicion is that if they're going to be effective they ought to be thinking about clearing the mind, so that they can just focus on what they need to do. Being clear about what their intention is. What the game plan is. And also accessing all of the skills and drills that they've been working on for years. They ought to be thinking, 'What quality of mind can I bring into this activity which will allow me to perform optimally?'

HARRIS: Should that be the key, though—not, 'How can I play to win,' necessarily, but 'How can I play my best?'

MUMFORD: Winning happens after a period of time. In basketball, for example, after 48 minutes. So you can focus on winning, but you have to be more focused on taking care of the present moment. If you perform each moment well, the results will take care of themselves. If you're focusing on results, then energy is being taken away from the activity that you're engaged in. Maybe before the game you can have the intention of winning and understanding what it takes to win, but it's more effective, in my experience, to be clear about what you need to do and what the team needs to win, and then go on out and perform it. If you're thinking about winning awards or about whether you're doing well or not, those things actually create a situation where you don't do well, because your mind is somewhere else. Your mind is not engaged in the activity. Any distraction is taking energy away, so you may only be operating on a couple of cylinders rather than all the cylinders.

HARRIS: As a spectator, you see that so often. You can have a game where things are going very well for one team and then maybe the other team scores a couple of times, and you can literally see the players start to lose their confidence.

MUMFORD: That's right. Absolutely. Confidence is a momentary thing. If you feel yourself lose confidence, you can maybe recite an affirmation or remember times when you were confident, and you can get it back. A lot of times we try to do something to get it back. Sometimes that works, and sometimes that's a setup to fail even more. Yogi Berra said 90 percent of baseball is mental and the other half is physical. That says it all. It really is mental. A lot of these folks have the same skill level, or they have the same

P R E S E N T

"You can focus on winning, but you have to be more focused on taking care of the present moment. If you perform each moment well, the results will take care of themselves."

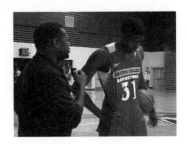

physiques or physical talent, but it's the ability to direct and control that talent that either allows that talent to manifest itself, or actually prevents the talent from being displayed.

HARRIS: And at the very elite levels, the difference between one team or another, or one individual or the other, can be very, very small.

MUMFORD: Absolutely, physically; but mentally, the difference can be huge.

HARRIS: You were on the floor with the Chicago Bulls for the last game of the '98 championship. What happened? It was a pretty amazing couple of minutes.

MUMFORD: Yes, it was quite amazing because it looked as if the Utah Jazz were in control of the game. Scotty Pippen was injured so he was playing sparingly, and wasn't able to be as active offensively or defensively as he would have liked. So it was what we call crunch time, and in my view of things everybody was playing well, but Michael was in the zone. He sort of took over the game.

HARRIS: How could you tell that's what he was doing?

MUMFORD: Well, just by the way he was doing things. Just by the way he seemed to be aware of what was going to happen before it happened. For instance, he scored the last eight points. There were maybe 23 seconds left. Karl Malone had the ball and Michael stripped him of the ball, and then he drove down and he scored. He didn't call time out. He assessed things. He talked afterward about being in the zone, but he seems to be in the zone more than most. It's not unusual for him to take over a game or for him to get into that place, but you could see he was playing on a different level from the other players.

HARRIS: It really is something you can see.

MUMFORD: Yes, you can see it. And you can feel it. When he scored that last basket and made it 87-86, it was like the energy of the whole place changed. It was like taking the air out of a bubble, because those fans in Utah were very loyal, and they were not pleasant to listen to, if you were on the other team. They were on the edge of winning. They were actually up by a point with less than 24 seconds left. Basically, they didn't have to score. They could have just held the ball. But they were going in to score, and they were about to score when Michael just went in, and he seemed to be one step ahead of everyone. You could see that by his behavior, by his play.

HARRIS: Is this something that he does very consciously? Or is this something that he's gotten better at since you've been working with the team?

MUMFORD: You'd have to ask him that. But one thing you notice about Michael, he has tremendous concentration. He works hard. He's able to find challenges for himself. Sometimes the more clarity he can have, the more he can train his mind to drop into those levels of concentration. My sense is, as you get older and you have less energy, you really need your mind, because you don't have the same stamina or the ability to jump and physically do all the things you used to do. I would say he's also much better because he knows how to use his skill and how to take advantage of the other team. So his perception, his clarity of what's going on and how to respond to it has increased. As he is more mindful, he'll be more effective. He's getting older. He's not supposed to be getting better. But somehow he is getting better all the time. And I think that has to do with the mental training.

HARRIS: We were talking a second ago about that very exciting last game against the Jazz last year, and it occurred to me as you were talking about how important intention is in terms of focus. Chances are, as Michael Jordan grabbed the ball he wasn't thinking, 'Oh my gosh, we've only got a few seconds left. I've got to do this or we're going to lose.'

MUMFORD: I can guarantee it wasn't that. Basically, knowing how much time is left and what the score is, you go down with the intention of trying to get the turnover and then coming back and scoring. He was in the moment, so he knew what to do.

HARRIS: What would have happened, do you think, if he had been worried? If he had allowed himself to think about whether it was going to work or not?

MUMFORD: Well, being inactive with very little time left in the game would give the defense a chance to react to him and recover. It's sort of like Tai Chi. You use the other person's energy against them, so when you see the opening you take it. You take advantage of the moment. It's the same in martial arts. You don't have time to think about it. You just train yourself, and you practice over a long period of time, so when the situation arises there's no thinking. It's just going down and taking care of business.

HARRIS: As opposed to worrying about it.

MUMFORD: As opposed to worrying about it. Just forming the intention and letting the body do it.

Quest for the Zone

The Zone—that place of deep concentration and seemingly effortless ability, a moment in time when time itself seems to slow down—is so elusive that athletes and others often bog down in the attempt to describe it.

"It's like playing in slow motion," one will say. Or, "It's when I can sense what will happen next and be there ahead of time, almost without knowing how I got there. I'm so calm and so focused, it's like everything is coming together all at once. But if I stop to acknowledge it, that breaks the spell and it's gone."

Acknowledgement of the zone is part of a growing awareness that peak perform-ance in sports encompasses more than perfect execution by a well-trained body. Only in the past 15 years or so have sports psychologists begun to define playing in the zone as a special state of focused awareness, an experience in which mind and body seem to be working together in perfect harmony.

Whether you're a weekend warrior or an elite athlete, you know it when you're there. It's getting there that can be maddeningly difficult.

Meditation and visualization techniques are often used in the attempt to reach it. Ironically, however, the harder you try, the harder it can be to get there. Gritting your teeth and muttering to yourself, "Relax and concentrate!" before an athletic event is almost sure to push you in the opposite direction. It happens when it hap-pens, some experts shrug, and trying too hard keeps it from happening at all.

There are some pointers they offer, however, including:

- Remember why you took up the sport in the first place: presumably, for the sheer enjoyment of it. Success and devotion often go hand in hand.

- Be open to the idea that you can find yourself in the zone. Invite it in, without trying to force it.

- Focus on what you want to have happen, without being concerned about the outcome. As you shoot, if you're worried about missing the target, chances are you will. If, on the other hand, you can take a wholehearted delight in the per-fection of the moment...you could find yourself in the zone with ease.

When you do, savor it as the gift it is. Like your first kiss, your baby's first step, or any other transcendent moment that you want to freeze and hold in your memory banks forever, a visit to the zone—however brief—is one of life's peak experiences.

HARRIS: I want to ask you about the coach of the Chicago Bulls, Phil Jackson. What's it been like to work with him?

MUMFORD: It's been quite a wonderful experience, because Phil has a reverence and a deep respect for what it means to be a human being and how to access a higher power, you might say. He's always looking to help the guys be better. He understands people. He understands how to get people to relate together in a collective way, as well as how to get them to exhibit their best individual selves.

HARRIS: Presumably he thought it was important that you come in and work with the team. Was it a hard sell, do you think? Was there any resistance from team members wondering, 'Who's this guy coming to talk to us about mind/body stuff?'

MUMFORD: When I started working with them back in '93, it was a big crisis because Michael had just retired. It would have been a little strange if I were to go in and just try to teach them to meditate. But when I talked to them about the benefits of having the mind and body in sync, or about being in the zone, they can relate to that moment that's different from other moments. They want to know, how does that happen? And is it possible for us to have more of those moments? So when I talk about those types of things, I get their interest, and when their interest is there, they're willing to try it. If they can have an experience, just a moment of what it's like, then that will speak for itself. All they have to do is deal with the goals that they have and the best way to attain them.

HARRIS: Maybe they were ready to hear it at that point because Michael was gone.

MUMFORD: My guess is that because there's so much respect for Phil, they were willing to do it. They assumed he would not bring someone in or

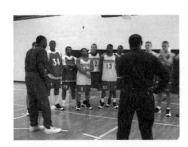
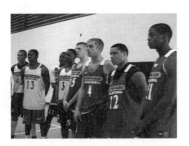
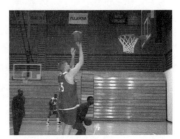

introduce them to something that wouldn't be helpful. They were used to him being a little bit different than most coaches. One word to describe the team would be teachable. In spite of the fact that they've been world champions so many times, they're always willing to look at things, be open, and continue to learn.

HARRIS: Do you ever have a player come to you and say, 'You know what? I tried what you said and it was amazing.'

MUMFORD: Yes. I've had those experiences with different players where they can see that it was beneficial to do this.

HARRIS: Are they surprised?

MUMFORD: I think they're surprised to some degree, but on another level I think they kind of know it's natural. When we have that experience of being fully in the moment, it feels right. It's exciting. Then the question is: can you keep doing it? And can you keep doing it without looking for those moments? Because looking for those moments will prevent you from having them. I would say that when they get a taste for it, that's enough to keep them interested.

HARRIS: So it becomes one of those times when you smack your forehead and say, 'So *that's* what it was.'

MUMFORD: Yes. And sometimes it takes years of doing it before you realize, 'Oh, that's what he's talking about,' or, 'This is what's possible.' Some of it is faith. When you have enough experiences of it, then you develop a conviction. I'm not ready to say that a lot of people on the team have a conviction at this point. But they have faith.

HARRIS: Is there a role for spirituality in here, too? Do you think that the athletes who feel some level of spiritual connection, whatever that might be, that it's helpful to them in how they perform athletically?

M O M E N T

"When we have that experience of being fully in the moment, it feels right. It's exciting. Then the question is: can you keep doing it? And can you keep doing it without looking for those moments? Because looking for those moments will prevent you from having them."

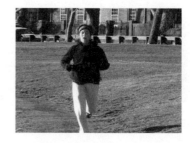

MUMFORD: I would say bringing spirit into any situation would be helpful. If you're talking about a creative energy, that sort of thing. If you're talking about being at peace with yourself, being at peace with your teammates, being at peace with the coaching staff or with your family, even if it's just a moment, that's extremely helpful. If you want to talk about spirituality in the sense of feeling connected to ourselves and other people, it's very important. When you talk to ex-players, what they miss about the game, besides performing and being out in front of all the folks, what they seem to miss most is the camaraderie of their teammates and being connected with a lot of people working toward a shared goal. The word spiritual can be very confusing at times. If you look at spirit in the sense of feeling connected with others and yourself, then I would say that spirituality is extremely helpful.

HARRIS: You also worked with the Bulls' Steve Kerr when he had some problems with injuries. How did your training help him recover?

MUMFORD: A lot of it is getting the physical therapy and allowing the injury to heal, but how you approach that whole situation can make a big difference. For instance, if you approach it like, 'Okay, I'm not playing. I have this free time. How am I going to use it? How am I going to relate to my injury? What's the best way for me to use my time so that when I get out on the court or when I go back to work I'll be able to perform effectively?' And I say, when people really are able to accept that they're injured and they're not playing, then a lot is possible in terms of being clear about what your intentions are, and the best way to bring those intentions into reality. For example, if you're injured and you're thinking about how this is your free-agency year and you don't have a contract for next year, you start thinking, 'What's this going to do to my marketing potential? What if somebody steps up and takes my job?' You can start worrying about all the things that can happen. And that energy, worrying about it, is creating tension and tightness in the body. It may even be setting you up to fail after you've healed physically, because that tension is going to impact your ability to go out and perform and do well. Or, you could use this time as a blessing in disguise: 'I have time to spend with my family. I have time to look at what's right in my life and appreciate the fact that I am playing, and I'm playing with this team. I can use this time to get to know myself better and learn how to be more in the moment.' That's very different. Steve used that situation to his benefit and says that it helped him to get in touch with himself and his family, as well as appreciating the gift of being able to practice mindfulness.

HARRIS: What would you say total consciousness is for an athlete?

CONSCIOUSNESS

MUMFORD: Total consciousness would be the experience of having your mind totally involved and absorbed in the activity that you're doing. Whether you're lifting weights or running laps or whatever it is, you're doing whatever the activity is. Your mind is totally focused on what you're doing without distracting thoughts, without worrying about how you're doing. There would be an absence of self-consciousness, so that you would actually lose yourself in the activity. That's the only thing you're thinking about. That's the only thing you're focused on.

HARRIS: What do you do, personally, to reinforce your own mindfulness?

MUMFORD: I practice sitting meditation, and I do a lot of stretching, a lot of moving meditation, Tai Chi, Qi Gong. I also study. I read books. I try to be aware of what my intentions are, what my motivations are, what my goals are; also what kind of belief systems I seem to be operating under. I question everything and put it under the microscope. If it's working, I keep it. If it leads to more wholeness for me, I keep doing it, and if not, I don't. A lot of it is just bringing my full mind into whatever activity I'm engaged in, and being clear about what I think I need to do.

HARRIS: I just have one more question. Let's say it's time out in the last seconds of a big game. The players and the coaches and everybody come to the bench. What do you tell them?

MUMFORD: I don't tell them anything, because I do my work outside of the realm of the actual game situation, and the coaches take over from there. My experience is just by them seeing me, knowing I'm there, they remember: 'George is here. Be mindful. Breathe.' They have to be focused on what they're doing. But I hope that they're reminded to breathe in and breathe out, and to go out there with as much of their mind engaged as they can.

"Total consciousness is...doing whatever the activity is. Your mind is totally focused on what you're doing without distracting thoughts, without worrying about how you're doing."

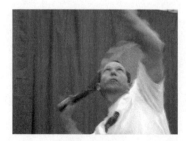

13 MINDFUL PARENTING: RAISING HAPPY, HEALTHY KIDS

I once was given a little pocket-sized book filled with sayings by and about women. One quote in particular has stayed with me ever since. "Making a decision to have a child," according to Elizabeth Stone, "means giving your heart permission to walk around outside your body."

Ah, yes. Like most of the rest of us, I had no idea what I was getting into when I had my son 12 years ago: how exciting, exhilarating, exhausting, exasperating, and totally all-encompassing the experience would be. Now, whenever a friend announces she's pregnant and turns a trusting face to me as an older mom, someone who has presumably learned from her mistakes, I usually smile and say, "It's the hardest you'll ever work, and it's the most fun you'll ever have."

I do believe that parenthood is both. The problem is, it all goes too fast. One minute you're burping an adorable infant, the next you're spending an anxious night at the bedside of a cranky and feverish toddler. Two more blinks of an eye, and you're being besieged for permission to let him go get pizza with his pals after school, and already starting to worry about what happens when he learns to drive.

I wish I had known then what I know now. Don't we all. One thing I have come to understand, though—even before Myla and Jon Kabat-Zinn wisely pointed it out—our children probably teach us more than we teach them. For one thing, they already know how to be happy. They've mastered the skill of being furious with us one minute, then, with remarkable speed, they're able to turn the page and move on. And they know how to greet each day as the gift that it is, filled with the promise of more adventures to come.

In this chapter, you'll find more good advice on how we can appreciate what our children do for us, as well as how we can be better parents to them.

JON AND MYLA KABAT-ZINN

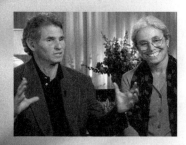

Jon and Myla Kabat-Zinn are the authors of *Everyday Blessings: The Inner Work of Mindful Parenting*, a book on how the practice of mindfulness can improve relationships between parents and their children. Jon Kabat-Zinn, Ph.D., is the founder and director of the Stress Reduction Clinic at the University of Massachusetts Medical Center. He is known throughout the world for his work in using mindfulness meditation to reduce chronic pain and stress-related disorders. His other books include *Wherever You Go, There You Are: Mindfulness Meditation in Everyday Life,* and *Full Catastrophe Living: Using the Wisdom of Your Body and Mind to Face Stress.* Myla Kabat-Zinn, B.S.N., R.N., has worked as a childbirth educator and birthing assistant. She is the former co-director of Birth Day, a Boston-area childbirth education organization. They are the parents of three children, ages 15, 19, and 23.

HARRIS: Do you feel that you've been successful as parents?

JON: I'm not sure that you ever feel that you're successful as a parent, but I think relatively speaking, the proof is in the pudding. It's how the children are, and it's constantly changing. It always has an element of struggle and uncertainty. Our work is about 'mindful parenting', which doesn't mean perfect parenting. It means doing the best that you can.

HARRIS: We assume that most parents, if not every parent, wants to do the right thing, wants to raise a wonderful child, wants to have a warm and loving atmosphere at home. How is mindful parenting different from what any loving parent would want to do?

MYLA: What we're talking about is a kind of intentional practice of mindfulness. If we don't bring a certain intentionality into our daily lives with our children, very often we find ourselves reacting automatically to situations in ways that are not necessarily helpful or healthy. Making it an intentional practice allows us to work with awareness in a way that allows us to experience being more conscious, more present, and more appropriate in our responses.

HARRIS: Can you give me some examples?

JON: I think it's very easy to be tuned out when you're preoccupied with your own life and to not pick up on the beauty of the present moment, especially with children. They encapsulate vitality and aliveness. They're captured by virtually everything in their world. One can easily not pick up on that. Depending on their age, of course, and depending on the circumstances, there are thousands of opportunities to tune in to your children, to try to drop in and see through their eyes, to experience alongside of them what they're experiencing in some way, to actually share their lives.

HARRIS: And that begins very early on. I'm struck by how much you try to see the world from the child's point of view. For example, you ask whether a baby would rather be in a stroller, or wrapped in their mom or dad's arms?

MYLA: If we start to see things from our children's point of view, it's a very different view. We've evolved over thousands and thousands of years, and for thousands of years, babies slept with their parents. They were held all the time, and we evolved, in some ways, to be in those situations. That's what babies need. Now we're living in an age where the relationships are very disembodied. It's only since the industrial revolution that we've really started to separate from babies so early. Between kids spending time at the computer and watching TV, and babies being put in carriages and baby seats, there's very little holding, very

INTENTIONALITY

"If we don't bring a certain intentionality into our daily lives with our children, very often we find ourselves reacting automatically to situations in ways that are not necessarily helpful or healthy."

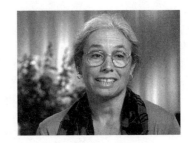

little touching. Children are starting to experience the world in very disembodied ways. I think that it's a real grounding for children, for babies, for toddlers to be held. It grounds them in the present moment. It grounds them in terms of their relationships, and it also gives them and the parent tremendous pleasure, which we're denying ourselves when we don't do that.

JON: That's what mindfulness allows you to do: to be in the present moment. Mindfulness means moment-to-moment, non-judging awareness. It's easy to talk about and very difficult to do, because so much of the time we're off someplace else, but we can bring ourselves back and really be in that moment. Touch is not simply with the body but also with one's heart, being able to embrace a child in your heart even when the child is doing something that you don't like, which is the most difficult time to do it.

HARRIS: How do you cultivate that? Is it simply a matter of being aware of what's going on right under your nose?

JON: Yes, and your awareness of how you want to judge it.

MYLA: You might think you're present in that moment when you're putting your child to bed, and then the next minute you're thinking about the next day, you're already worrying about what you have to accomplish, and you lose something. Bringing your attention back into the present moment can be a tremendously powerful exercise and endeavor. That's what we're talking about.

JON: And learning to be still a little bit, instead of immediately jumping onto the next thing. When you're waking a child up in the morning, if you're in a hurry, you'll transmit that to the child along with a good deal of anxiety. The same thing with putting a child to bed at night, or having a conversation with a child, or at any of the junctures during the day when there's contact. It can be either automatic and mechanical, or it can be heartful and mindful, and we can make those choices literally from moment to moment. The curious thing

HOLDING

"I think it's a real grounding for children, for babies, for toddlers to be held. It grounds them in the present moment. It grounds them in terms of their relationships, and it also gives them and the parent tremendous pleasure, which we're denying ourselves when we don't do that."

is, when we do, it not only feeds the children, it deeply feeds us. It's almost as if you could turn parenting into a profound spiritual practice, without ever meditating in the full lotus posture or anything like that. You can see your children as profound spiritual teachers about life and what's important.

HARRIS: I want to expand on that thought a bit, because many people think that the job of the parent is to be the teacher, but maybe it's the other way around. What have you learned from your children?

MYLA: We can learn a lot from our children, and it's very different at different ages. When they're babies, they teach us unconditional love. Children are wonderfully forgiving. When they're little, they are so happy to see us. One minute, they can be angry, and the next minute, they're just starting fresh. In some ways, watching them let go of their anger teaches us that we can let go of our anger and start fresh again. As children get older, they teach us other things. With teenagers, I think the biggest lesson we learn from them is acceptance, trying to work with accepting who they are, and the ways in which they express themselves. Sometimes we don't like the way they express themselves as teenagers, but we still love them.

JON: That opens up our own hearts, as we realize that it's not our job as parents to force them to be exactly as we would like them to be—as hard as that is, sometimes, to admit. Parenting is an incredible opportunity to be attentive to the jewels that fall out of their mouths and out of their lives. There are lots of wonderful little anecdotes that we hear from parents all over the country, those moments where you really see through the child's eyes, and you begin to realize the enormity of the learning process to become a fully embodied human being. Like a child saying to her mother, when her mother is driving in traffic and getting quite upset, and she hears a little voice from the car seat saying,

F
O
R
G
I
V
I
N
G

"Children are wonderfully forgiving...one minute they can be angry, and the next minute, they're just starting fresh. In some ways, watching them let go of their anger teaches us that we can let go of our anger and start fresh again."

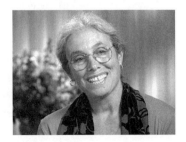

'Mommy, are you angry?' The mother says, 'Yes, I am angry. Here we are stuck in traffic, and we have to be somewhere.' And the child says, 'But, Mommy, we're traffic, too.' Little remembrances, little reminders. Those happen all the time.

HARRIS: We were talking a moment ago about trying to quiet that internal dialogue that many of us have in our heads. Even when we're trying to be with our kids, we're thinking, 'I have this phone call to make, and do I have orange juice for tomorrow, and do I have the makings for the school lunch,' and all of that. Even when our children are babies, can they tell when we're really not there for them?

MYLA: Absolutely. Children are wonderful at being able to know when we're present and when we're not. If we have a kind of open communication with them, very often they tell us, 'Hey Mom, come back. You're not here.' They really learn from us, from our being. If we can be more present with them, they learn a certain sense of being present in the world. It also is a feeling of being honored. You know when you're with somebody, and you really feel that they're giving you their full attention. In a sense, it's a gift to you. Obviously, there are going to be times in the day where we can't give our attention to our children. That's fine, but too often that becomes the mode of being. Bringing mindfulness back, bringing our attention to our breath, grounding ourselves in our body, we bring ourselves back into the present moment, and that becomes a gift. The child feels we're there, we're really listening, and we're really paying attention.

So often we think we have to give our children tangible gifts. We're very oriented in our society to buying; that's the way we give our children love. But very often what is most meaningful to children is the gift of our presence. In workshops that we've given, when we've asked people to talk about moments when they felt truly seen by another person in their family, it was often something very simple, like having their hands in the dirt with their grandfather, out in the garden. That moment stays with them their whole lives. They felt his really being there for them.

P R E S E N C E

"So often we think we have to give our children tangible gifts...but very often what is most meaningful to children is the gift of our presence."

Adventure Game Theater

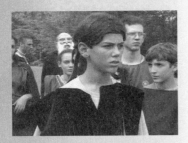

P R O F I L E

The Adventure Game Theater is one of those experiences for which words seem inadequate. Brought to the Omega Institute in upstate New York 12 years ago by its creators, Howard Moody and Brian Allison, it is a colorful blend of fantasy, improvisation, and discovery—and all of it, for teenagers only.

"In other cultures, in other times, there have been much more clear rites of passage for kids," says Omega co-founder Elizabeth Lesser, who embraced the idea with enthusiasm from the moment it was brought to her. "It's very confusing to be a teenager today. What this program does is give a sense of ritual to the stage that these teenagers are going through."

From its beginning early in Omega's annual "Family Week" through the days and nights that follow, each "adventure" has its own story line that is then brought to life by as many as 100 young people, aged 12 to 18. Each story is wildly imaginative, with oracles, healers, wizards and wise women, gods and goddesses, merchants and thieves. Players can be as inventive as they please; costumes, masks, and makeup help add excitement to the mix. Swordplay—with swords made of foam—is a perennial favorite, especially with the younger teens. In this version, what counts most is not the skill or ferocity of the fighter, but whether their opponent "dies" with dignity. Instant resurrection then enables the vanquished player to come back as a new character.

"It's like being in your own movie," says Moody, who, along with Allison, first came up with the idea as a vehicle for adults. After its introduction, however, teenagers loved the program so much that it has been theirs ever since. "We prepare for several days, so that by Wednesday night when the story actually begins, the kids have the

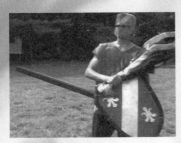

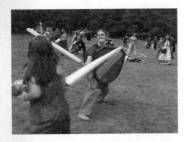

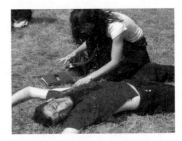

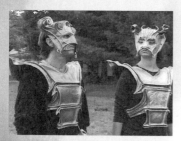 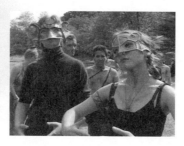 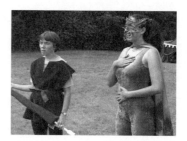

feeling that they're about to enter a wonderful fantasy world, a magical place that might exist on another planet or in another dimension. In an eight-hour story, many of these players are living out a whole mythic fantasy, living deeply through their characters."

The larger message of coexistence and peaceful conflict resolution is cleverly disguised by the playful nature of the adventure. If an AGT player goes home with a new understanding of the challenges in getting along with other people—how to balance the enthusiasm of the 12-year-olds with the more reasoned approach of the 18-year-olds, for example—so much the better. But it's never imposed on them in a way that seems heavy-handed.

"Over the years, we've found that using this theater form and allowing the kids to so freely and creatively express themselves brings a very deep sense of community. As kids come back year after year, the community deepens," Moody said.

What the players remember is how much fun it all was, in addition to what it taught them.

"You have a character that you've been given by someone else and you become that character," recalls 17-year-old Terre Unité Parker, a college freshman and an AGT veteran. "It's not like pretending; it's like you truly feel in your heart whatever's happening to that character. I've cried over somebody I lost, I've been completely joyful about saving some group, and when you're in those moments, you lose yourself inside that character. And then when I put that character away and come back to who I really am, I see how much I've learned from being that other person, and I become so much stronger that way.

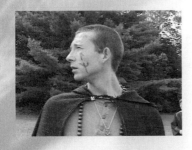

"Now that I've played every character imaginable, I have so many different aspects of myself that I've realized I can still use. The character shows me qualities about myself that I haven't discovered before, who I really am inside—that I can be all those different things. It's so wonderful to realize that."

HARRIS: You've written, 'Love is expressed in how you pass the bread and how you say good morning and not just the trip to Disney World.' How do you remember that, though? It sounds simple, but it's easy to forget.

JON: It's very easy to forget. The mind goes here and the mind goes there, and we experience a lot of turmoil with our emotions as well. When we're feeling threatened or overwhelmed, or anxious because of one thing or another, it can spill out all over the place in terms of hurriedness, time urgency, irritability. All sorts of things spill out at the breakfast table or when you come home at the end of a long day. You're exhausted, out of sorts and thinking about a million different things, and you brush off your children in one way or another, or your spouse, for that matter. How do you remember? You keep bringing your attention back to the present moment. Why? Because it's the only moment that you're ever going to be alive in. It's this one.

You can be awake in a fraction of a second. You can be kindhearted in a fraction of a second. You can let go of your irritability, or your annoyance, or your anxiety. It requires a certain kind of discipline. I like to think of it as strengthening a muscle. If you want to grow this muscle, you put a weight in your hand, and you work against the resistance of the weight. Up, down; up, down. The mind goes off, you bring it back. The mind goes off again, you bring it back again.

In that way, you're actually growing a muscle that is of tremendous value in terms of your own healing as a person, your own transformation, and the opening of your heart and mind. It's the cultivation of wisdom. It's the cultivation of self-knowledge and self-compassion, and it opens the heart to other people. So it's of tremendous benefit to do that, but it is a discipline, and you have to be somewhat intentional about it. It's an act of love, actually, to accord yourself your own moments while you're still alive to experience them. Otherwise, 30 years can go by, and you say, 'What happened?'

HARRIS: You hear a lot of people lament, 'Gosh, my kids are all grown up,' or, 'He's 10, now, or 15, or she's eight already, and it seems like just last week that she was in diapers. How did it happen so fast?' It does make you think about how quickly time goes by, and how important it is to pay attention.

MYLA: Our lives are getting more and more crazy and hectic, and time is moving faster and faster. I think we all feel that. The wonderful aspect of being in the present moment is that it's timeless. I don't have a formal meditation practice, but the few times I experienced formal meditation when we were doing workshops, I really saw what that does in terms of slowing time down. It's a wonderful thing for parents to take the time, even for 10 minutes, to just sit.

JON: Even for 30 seconds. We're not suggesting that to be a mindful parent you have to be a meditator in any kind of formal sense. What we're saying is that anybody can cultivate mindfulness right through everything you're doing. So at the breakfast table, what's the tone in your voice when you're asking for something? Are you making eye contact when you say goodbye? Are you screaming? There are so many different moments in the day with children of any age, even talking on the phone to grown-up children far away. You can be fully present, or you can be half present, and it's felt immediately. It influences the long-term qualities of the relationship.

HARRIS: It also makes me wonder, if we're tuning them out when they're little, is that why they often tune us out as they get older?

MYLA: As children get older, sometimes they need to tune us out. That's part of growing up and leaving home. But when they value the relationship—and that's really what this work is all about, valuing the relationship—then I think

R E L A T I O N S H I P

"There are so many different moments in the day with children of any age, even talking on the phone to grown-up children far away. You can be fully present, or you can be half present, and it's felt immediately. It influences the long-term qualities of the relationship."

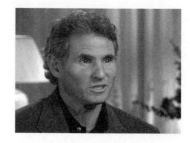

that carries through as they get older. There's a certain sense of honoring each other. As Jon said, even if it's in a phone call with our older children, it's amazing the difference that can make in the quality of the relationship.

HARRIS: But how do you remember that in the heat of the moment?

JON: That's where the discipline comes in. How do you go up to the plate with 40,000 fans screaming at you, and you've got everything on the line to hit the 62nd home run of the season? What do you do with your mind? You've got to watch this baseball coming at you at 90 miles an hour. You have to be present. You have to pay attention. We love to watch someone else do it, but we can do it ourselves at our own level, at our own pace in our lives. That's why we call it inner work. But the payoff, the value of doing something like this, is huge over the life span. It's almost like walking out of a black and white movie into a color movie. It's like breathing life into your own life, and that is its own gift and its own joy.

HARRIS: You also talk about 'honoring and acknowledging the sovereignty of the child.' Many people would look at a phrase like that and ask, 'What are you saying here, that anything they want to do is fine? We're just going to let them run wild?'

MYLA: No, that's not what we're saying. Honoring who that child is means looking beneath the surface of their behavior. Very often, we get caught up in the surface. 'Oh my God, she wants to get her nose pierced,' or, 'She wants to dye her hair purple,' or, 'My two-year-old is biting.' If you get caught up in that, you forget to look beneath the surface. Like with a two-year-old biting: two-year-olds bite sometimes when they can't express themselves. So you say, 'No, you can't bite,' but you're not saying, 'You're a terrible kid because you're biting.' You're seeing it with the awareness that, sometimes, two-year-olds bite when

P A Y O F F

"You have to be present. You have to pay attention. But the payoff, the value of doing something like this, is huge over the life span. It's almost like walking out of a black and white movie into a color movie. It's like breathing life into your own life."

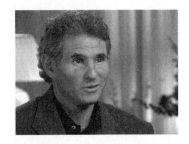

they're frustrated and they can't say what they want. It's the same with older children. Setting limits, or having very clear values and standing firm when it's hardest for us to do that, takes a lot of energy. But that's the way we really show our love and our honor of their sovereignty. Sometimes it's a huge struggle, where the easy way would be to say, 'Sure, do what you want.' That's not what we call honoring the sovereignty of the child.

JON: A lot of it will stretch our envelope. We're continually being stretched. It's the yoga of parenting. 'Oh, you've been stretched this far? Okay, now we're going to stretch you a little further.' That's what children do. They stretch our limits. They are always challenging, and I want to be clear about the agony of parenting. There are moments when we feel like we're the worst possible parents in the world, that no matter how mindful we are, it's just a disaster, that it's going to all collapse, that our children are incredibly vulnerable and potentially in situations that make us cringe. This is part of the work. It's not like, 'Oh, if we were doing it better, that wouldn't happen,' and this is a very important thing to realize. Life is real. It's not that if you do this in some formulaic way, everything will just work out. There are times that we go into deep experiences of darkness, where we worry deeply about our children. All parents do, but you can bring awareness to that, too. In the most upsetting moments lie the root and the seed of transformation. Mindfulness is the cultivation of emotional intelligence. Families that honor emotions grow children who are competent in the vast range of different emotional situations, and don't get hijacked or railroaded by emotional storms to the point where they become really self-destructive. Or less so, anyway.

HARRIS: You've written that being a parent requires a certain amount of spiritual discipline. What do you mean by that?

JON: I guess what I'm saying is that parenting could be seen as a spiritual discipline, but one would have to choose to see it that way. Otherwise, it will go right by you. If you understand spiritual discipline, it's an opportunity to work on yourself, to do a certain kind of inner work. We're good at working on cars, working on boats, working at the office, working for institutions, doing all sorts of outer work. Inner work is the work of coming to understand yourself more fully as a human being, inquiring what it means to be fully human in your body, in your life as it's unfolding. Very often, people will go to spiritual centers for that, or they'll pray, or they'll do a whole range of disciplines to cultivate the heart, to cultivate a more spiritual orientation, a more forgiving, more loving, and more caring orientation. What we're saying is, there's no better environment for that kind of work to happen than in the family.

We have children that could be seen as little live-in Zen masters, so to speak, parachuted into our lives. They're inevitably going to push all our buttons, question all our assumptions, demand that we expand beyond our limits, and we have different ways that we could respond to that. One would be to get very tough and try to control everything because we're bigger, and we know everything. Or we could use it as an opportunity to grow, ourselves, and to realize we don't know everything. We might pretend we know everything, but we don't. We're lucky if we know who we are. It's a wonderful opportunity within family life and within parenting to use all of these occasions as the fuel for doing this inner work of inquiry, of cultivating empathy, cultivating acceptance, and honoring our own true being. There's no one formula for doing this; there's no one right way to parent.

HARRIS: You also write about being able to back off and ask yourself the question, 'What's really important here?' Why is that the question?

MYLA: Because so often we forget what's most important. We get caught up in our fears, our anxieties, and we lose sight of what is most important. Very often, the only way we can get to that question is to both see things from our child's point of view and also be aware of our own feelings. In the process of stopping a moment and saying, 'What's really going on here? What's really needed here? What's this like for my child? What's this like for me?'—sometimes that points you to something completely different. Very often, we get caught up in the least important thing, because that's where our fear takes us. So that question really allows us to choose a more appropriate and healthy response to very difficult situations, the ones that push our buttons the most, and often bring up responses that are replaying tapes from our own childhood. Many times, our automatic reactions are things we learned when we were very little. It's amazing how affected we are by our own experience as children. If we don't look at that, we can find ourselves doing things that later we regret. Sometimes we may even go down that path, but if we can bring awareness to what happened, next time perhaps we'll choose a different way.

HARRIS: I would imagine there's not a parent in America who hasn't said to him or herself at least once, 'I can't believe I did that. That's what my mother or father always did to me. I always swore that I would never do it with my own kids.'

JON: Absolutely. An initiation into parenthood is to realize that you used to say, 'I'd never do what my father did,' and then you wind up having a child, and then you're doing the exact same thing. You become your father. Maybe that's part of our own growing, to realize a certain humility that we're not all that different from our parents, and that our children, do what we will, are going to be who they are. Ultimately, the work is to honor that and not try to control the world beyond what our capacities are. Maybe if we collaborated with the world rather than trying to move it where we think it needs to be, we'd grow in our own hearts and souls.

HARRIS: I have to ask one last question, and that is, what will you say to your children one day about how you would like them to raise your grandchildren?

JON (laughing): We'll keep our mouths shut, I think.

MYLA: This kind of work is about not imposing our desires on our children. We haven't gotten there [being grandparents] yet, but I think it's a wonderful reminder that parenting is never over. Whether we have small children or grown children or whether we're grandparents, we're still parents, and the relationship is constantly changing. We're always renegotiating the agreements. When your child goes off to college, it's different from when your child graduates from college or goes off into the work world. Sometimes our children come home again, and we have to renegotiate. When our children get married, it's a whole other renegotiation, but the work of mindfulness is about meeting each moment freshly so it calls for something new. If we get stuck and treat our 30-year-old child the way we did our 20-year-old child, we're in big trouble.

JON: All I can say is that I truly feel blessed to have had the opportunity to be a father and to experience the many ways in which it's taught me about life that I would not have known otherwise. We have to, in some way, trust in the uniqueness and the integrity of each child to find their own way and to follow their own passion. Very often, the things that you don't like about what they're doing along the way, are things that they absolutely have to do in order to come into their own. There's a certain point at which we have to learn to let go, and if there's growing to be done, let our children do their growing, and let's continue to do ours.

RESOURCE SUPPLEMENT

From the editors of *New Age: The Journal for Holistic Living*

HOW TO CHOOSE AN ALTERNATIVE PRACTITIONER

Today, more options than ever are available for those who want to explore the promise of holistic healing methods. But these new options can be confusing. How do you sort through often unfamiliar therapies and credentials to find the best care? We asked some experts in the field of holistic health for their advice on how to be a smart consumer.

Explore your options while you are well. Don't wait until you are ill to find a practitioner you trust. You can make less rushed, more thoughtful decisions about practitioners when you are not distracted by the physical and emotional toll of an illness, notes Joan Borysenko, psychologist and cofounder of the Mind/Body Medical Institute at Beth Israel Deaconess Hospital.

Borysenko suggests that you set up a "get acquainted" visit with any practitioner whom you are considering. Though this kind of shopping around may cost you some money, it can prove well worth the investment: Many holistic practitioners will work with you over many years to help keep you well. And should you become ill, just knowing that there is already a trusted practitioner to turn to can greatly reduce your stress.

Do your homework. If you have a condition you would like to treat with holistic methods and you don't already have a practitioner or modality you prefer, how do you decide whether to turn to, say, an acupuncturist or a homeopath for care?

One place to start is through networking with friends and acquaintances who have had a similar condition and have obtained good results with a treatment or practitioner. Self-help groups organized around illnesses can also be helpful in this regard. Look through the holistic-health titles in bookstores, search the Internet for health-related online support groups, or attend conferences at holistic learning centers on health topics.

Don't be afraid to experiment. Finding a treatment regime that works for you can sometimes mean trying out a number of different healing methods. Says William J. Goldwag, M.D., a holistic doctor with a practice in Stanton, California: "What works for one person may not work for someone else with the same problem. A lot of any medical practice—Western or otherwise—is trial and error. You start someplace and end up somewhere else."

In the event of serious illness, get an adequate diagnosis. Even if you do plan on having your illness treated with herbs, massage, or some other holistic therapy, it's still a good idea to have serious symptoms first evaluated by someone who has had a thorough clinical training in diagnosis. Remember that receiving a diagnosis from a medical doctor doesn't mean that you have to follow his or her prescribed treatment—it's simply to give you information so that you can then make your own decisions about what course of treatment is right for you.

Investigate a practitioner's credentials. There's a wide variation in the background and training of holistic practitioners. Licensing regulations governing specific fields—where they exist at all—often vary from state to state. So it's important for you to inquire about a practitioner's background: Where and for how long did he or she train? Did that training include clinical experience, or was it done through the mail? Is the practitioner licensed or certified? What did that process entail? What conditions does the practitioner's training qualify him or her to treat? What conditions can't the practitioner treat? (Be cautious of someone who assures you that his or her method can unquestionably cure "everything.")

If you want more information about the quality of a practitioner's training, professional associations that govern specific fields often can offer an evaluation of a school or training program's reputation or provide a listing of practitioners who are officially certified or licensed.

Get clear about your treatment plan before you begin. Discuss what to expect from a treatment with a practitioner before you agree to it, recommends Alan Gaby, M.D., past president of the American Holistic Medical Association (AHMA). Among the points to go over with the practitioner: How many people have you treated with my condition? What percentage of the time do you have success in treating my condition? What are the possible adverse reactions or side effects of the treatment? How many visits will the treatment require? At what point is it reasonable to expect that I will feel better? How much will it cost? Are there any research reports or clinical studies to back up this treatment?

In evaluating responses, Gaby advises that you take the practitioner's tone as well as the content into account. "I would rather have a practitioner tell me that 30 percent of people experience side effects than one who brushes off my questions or gets defensive," he says.

Remember that you are in charge. At any time in the process, don't be afraid to stop a treatment if you don't feel that it is working for you. Don't worry about being a "bad patient" or hurting a practitioner's feelings: "The practitioner doesn't pay you; you pay the practitioner," says Dana Ullman, co-author of *Everybody's Guide to Homeopathic Medicines.* "So if this employee doesn't completely satisfy you, he or she should be replaced."

Trust your own impressions. Chemistry can be almost as important as credentials in finding the right practitioner. In a helpful brochure entitled "How to Choose a Holistic Health Practitioner," the AHMA offers some questions to consider when evaluating whether a practitioner is a good "fit" for you. Among them: Do you feel comfortable and cared for when you visit the office? Is your appointment time honored, or do you have to wait? How do you feel when you are in this environment? Is the practitioner accessible? Is the practitioner sensitive enough to place him or herself in your position regarding fears and anxieties about an illness or proposed treatment?

If you would like to compare your impressions with those of other patients, ask for references from the doctor's roll of patients. Or you might strike up a conversation at the magazine rack in the waiting room and ask other patients about their experiences.

What to do about Dr. Wrong. One *Time*/CNN poll found that 84 percent of respondents who visited an alternative practitioner would go back to one. But what should you do if you are dissatisfied with the treatment you have received? The first step in addressing your concerns may simply be a frank talk. If you have a serious complaint, you should complain at the state level to the board that issued the practitioner's license. For practitioners of modalities not licensed by the state, the procedure is less clear-cut. Try contacting professional associations for advice and follow-up.

A GUIDE TO HOLISTIC TREATMENTS

Bodywork and Massage Therapy

Practitioners use hands-on techniques to manipulate the bones, muscles, or other tissue.

Acupressure
Bodywork for Abuse Survivors
Bonnie Prudden Myotherapy
Breema Bodywork
Chiropractic
Conscious Bodywork
CranioSacral Therapy
Deep Tissue Bodywork
Hellerwork
Infant Massage
Jin Shin Do
Kripalu Bodywork
Massage Therapy
Muscular Therapy
Myofascial Release
Neuromuscular Therapy
Reflexology
Rolfing
Shiatsu
Soma Neuromuscular Integration
Structural Integration
Swedish Massage
Trigger Point/Myotherapy
Watsu (Water Shiatsu)

Counseling

Practitioners use verbal techniques to encourage psychological and emotional healing. Some counselors also incorporate movement, bodywork, and other techniques in their practices.

Astrology
Bioenergetics
Body-Mind Counseling
Body-Oriented Psychotherapy
Career/Life Counseling
Core Energetics
Expressive Therapies
Focusing
Gestalt Therapy
Guided Imagery
Hypnotherapy
Intuitive Arts
Music/Sound Therapies
Neuro-Linguistic Programming
Option Method
Past Life/Regression Therapies
Pathwork
Rebirthing
Spiritual/Shamanic Healing

Energy Therapies

Practitioners use their hands to redirect the flow of bodily energy, release energy blocks, or send healing energy.

AMMA Therapy
Barbara Brennan Healing Science
Energy Field Work
Healing Touch

Jin Shin Jyutsu
Ohashiatsu
Polarity Therapy
Reiki
Robert Jaffe Advanced Energy Healing
SHEN Therapy
Therapeutic Touch
Touch for Health
Vibrational Healing
Zero Balancing

Holistic Health
Practitioners use a variety of healing methods to treat a range of diseases or provide primary care.

Anthroposophic Medicine
Ayurvedic Medicine
Chinese Medicine
Holistic Dentistry
Holistic Medicine
Naturopathic Medicine
Osteopathic Medicine

Movement Therapies
Practitioners lead clients through movements, body-awareness exercises, and/or breathing exercises designed to improve their health.

Aikido
Alexander Technique
Body-Mind Centering
Dance/Movement Therapies
Feldenkrais Method/Awareness
    Through Movement
Gyrotonics
Kripalu Yoga

Ortho-Bionomy
Phoenix Rising Yoga Therapy
Pilates Method
Qi Gong (Chi-Kung)
Rosen Method
Rubenfeld Synergy Method
Tai Chi/Martial Arts
Trager Bodywork
Yoga

Natural Healing Therapies
Practitioners specialize in a certain modality or technique.

Acupuncture
Aromatherapy
Biofeedback
Breathwork
Chelation Therapy
Colon Therapy
Ear Candling
Fasting
Feng Shui
Flower Essences
Herbalism
Homeopathy
Iridology
Kinesiology/Applied Kinesiology
Macrobiotic Counseling
Magnetic Therapy

PAYING FOR YOUR CARE

If you use the services of a holistic health practitioner, can you expect your insurance to help pick up the tab? The answer is mixed. More and more health insurers are covering therapies that were once considered alternative but are now accepted as mainstream.

The alternative therapies most likely to be covered are those in relatively well-established fields: acupuncture, biofeedback, chiropractic, hypnotherapy, naturopathy, nurse-midwifery, and osteopathy. Of course, whether the treatment you use is covered or not depends on a number of variables: your policy, your insurance company, the credentials of the practitioner, and your state's licensing laws. Here's a quick look at how different forms of insurance handle alternative health:

HMOs

A 1995 survey of the nation's largest HMOs found that as many as 86 percent of them covered some type of alternative therapy. Kaiser Permanente, the nation's largest private HMO (800-464-4000), has provided acupuncture to its members for more than a decade; now its broad-based wellness program includes nutritional counseling, massage, meditation, acupressure, and behavioral medicine as well.

An alternative therapy may be more likely to be covered if it is practiced by a participating physician. If you can find a participating physician who is also an acupuncturist, for example, then his or her acupuncture services would probably be covered.

Non-HMOs

Christine Roche, author of *The Insurance Reimbursement Manual*, writes that, generally speaking, "Insurance companies pay only for the treatment of disorders or diseases diagnosed by a healthcare professional who is licensed to practice in his or her state." Thus, insurance that won't cover massage or bodywork performed for relaxation purposes may cover massage or bodywork prescribed by a medical doctor, chiropractor, or osteopath as part of a treatment program for a particular disease or disorder. Similarly, holistic-health services performed by an M.D. would be the easiest kind to get covered. In addition, some health plans now reimburse for services provided by licensed acupuncturists and naturopathic physicians.

Specialty Companies

A few insurance companies now specialize in plans that cover holistic-health therapies. Such companies include Alternative Health Insurance Services (800-966-8467), Mutual of Omaha (800-456-0228), and Oxford Health Plans (800-444-6222). Some of these insurers only operate in certain states.

Finally, remember that you can play an important role in getting insurance carriers to expand their coverage. The reason more insurers are beginning to cover alternative therapies is that a growing number of people have asked for such coverage.

GETTING RUBBED THE RIGHT WAY

So you've finally carved free an hour from your busy schedule and have made an appointment for your first massage. The last thing you want to do is make it a stressful experience. Here are six pointers that will help get the ooohhhs and aaahhhs flowing:

Be an informed consumer. After checking the bodyworker listings in the telephone book and other resources, ask your friends about any whom you're considering. After all, the most reliable form of advertising is word-of-mouth. If that doesn't narrow your choices enough, feel free to call the bodyworkers themselves and inquire if they offer the kind of massage you are looking for— a light, relaxing touch or deeper, more therapeutic strokes. Also, before you schedule a massage, be aware of some caveats for people with particular physical conditions. If you're pregnant, for instance, seek out someone who specializes in massage on pregnant women. And massage may be unsafe for people with some types of cancer, some circulatory ailments, some skin disorders, and other conditions. If you're in doubt, consult your physician.

Stake out your comfort zone. It's your massage, not the bodyworker's. Though he or she probably will ask some questions and set a few ground rules before the session, you also should assert yourself about which parts of your body need extra attention and which areas you don't want touched at all. (The genitals are off-limits in any legitimate massage, of course, but you may also be averse to having, say, your tender ankle worked on.) When it's time for you to get on the table, remove only as much clothing as you feel okay shedding. Some bodyworkers will specify that you should keep your underwear on and will drape your body with a sheet or towel, uncovering only the part being worked on; others will allow you to go buck naked. Don't be shy about insisting that you be covered, if that will make you more comfortable.

Your job is to do nothing. The bodyworker doesn't need your help in lifting your leg, arm, or head off the table for a manipulation. Think of this as a 60-minute vacation—a day on the beach, without getting all that sand between your toes. Feel free to space out or even doze off, relaxing in mind and muscle. If you'd prefer to make the massage a less passive experience, then try this: Visualize yourself as the bodyworker's hands, probing into your muscles, working all around your body. This will not only lull you into an almost hypnotic peacefulness but may give you newfound body awareness as well.

Stay in touch. Sure, you'll probably sink more deeply into the massage experience by lying quietly on the table rather than chatting about the weather. But don't let that stop you from speaking up if you want, say, more (or less) time spent on whatever body part is being worked on. More pressure. Less oil. Remember: Feedback held till the end of the massage will only benefit the next person on the bodyworker's table. The idea isn't to respond to every stroke; that'll prove distracting to both you and the bodyworker. However, if the bodyworker seems unresponsive to any of your feedback or insists that you just lie there quietly, you should assert yourself—or seek out another bodyworker next time.

Don't grit your teeth and bear it. This really could be included as part of the above tip, but it warrants being singled out because it addresses massage's most unpleasant topic: pain. Though the deeper work in a massage may cause some discomfort, pain is not what a massage is all about. Yet for some reason, people often are afraid to tell their bodyworkers to lighten up. Don't be a martyr, lying there silently repeating the mantra: "Please move on to the other leg soon. Please move on to the other leg soon." Forget the adage "no pain, no gain"; you have a lot to gain by speaking out against pain.

Remember to breathe. Pretty rudimentary advice, eh? Well, when you've just undressed and are lying on a table, waiting to be rubbed down with warm oil by a stranger, you may have a tendency to hold your breath. This will not enhance the massage experience, of course, since by holding your breath you're also holding your tension. Instead, try to breathe as deeply and consciously as you can; that'll give you the best chance of becoming fully relaxed. Even the pain caused by massaging deeply into a sensitive area can be alleviated by deepening the breath. So inhale, exhale, and enjoy.

THE WHOLE-SELF BOOKSHELF

Books by Body & Soul Experts

SARAH BAN BREATHNACH
Something More: Excavating Your Authentic Self (Warner Books, 1998)
Simple Abundance: A Daybook of Comfort and Joy (Warner Books, 1995)
The Simple Abundance Journal of Gratitude (Warner Books, 1996)

LIBBY BARNETT AND MAGGIE CHAMBERS
Reiki Energy Medicine: Bring the Healing Touch into Home, Hospital and Hospice
  (Healing Arts, 1996)

HERBERT BENSON, M.D.
Timeless Healing: The Power and Biology of Belief (Fireside, 1997; with Marg Stark)
*The Wellness Book: The Comprehensive Guide to Maintaining Health and Treating Stress-
  Related Illness* (Fireside, 1993; co-author, Eileen M. Stuart)
The Relaxation Response (Avon, 1976)

TERAH KATHRYN COLLINS
*The Western Guide to Feng Shui: Creating Balance, Harmony, and Prosperity in Your
  Environment* (Hay House, 1996)

LARRY DOSSEY, M.D.
Be Careful What You Pray for . . . You Just Might Get It (HarperCollins, 1998)
Prayer Is Good Medicine (HarperCollins, 1996)
Healing Words: The Power of Prayer and the Practice of Medicine (HarperCollins,
  1993)

DAVID EISENBERG, M.D.
Encounters with Qi: Exploring Chinese Medicine (W.W. Norton, 1995)

PEGGY HUDDLESTON
Prepare for Surgery, Heal Faster (Angel River, 1996)

PHIL JACKSON
Sacred Hoops: Spiritual Lessons of a Hardwood Warrior (Hyperion, 1996; with
  Hugh Delehanty)

JON KABAT-ZINN, Ph.D.
Wherever You Go, There You Are: Mindfulness Meditation in Everyday Life
  (Hyperion, 1994)
*Full Catastrophe Living: Using the Wisdom of Your Body and Mind to Face Stress, Pain,
  and Illness* (Dell, 1990)
Everyday Blessings: The Inner Work of Mindful Parenting (Hyperion, 1998; co-author,
  Myla Kabat-Zinn)

DHARMA SINGH KHALSA, M.D.
Brain Longevity: The Breakthrough Medical Program that Improves Your Mind and Memory (Warner Books, 1997)

RONNA KABATZNICK, Ph.D.
The Zen of Eating: Ancient Answers to Modern Weight Problems (Perigree, 1998)

MICHAEL LERNER, Ph.D.
Choices in Healing: Integrating the Best of Conventional and Complementary Approaches to Cancer (MIT Press, 1994)

CHRISTIANE NORTHRUP, M.D.
Women's Bodies, Women's Wisdom: Creating Physical and Emotional Health and Healing (Bantam Doubleday Dell, 1998).

STEPHAN RECHTSCHAFFEN, M.D.
Timeshifting: Creating More Time to Enjoy Your Life (Doubleday, 1997)

STELLA RESNICK, Ph.D.
The Pleasure Zone: Why We Resist Good Feelings & How to Let Go & Be Happy (Conari, 1997)

GENEEN ROTH
When You Eat at the Refrigerator, Pull Up a Chair: 50 Ways to Be Thin, Gorgeous, and Happy When You Feel Anything But (Hyperion, 1998)
Appetites: On the Search for True Nourishment (Plume, 1997)
Feeding the Hungry Heart: The Experience of Compulsive Eating (Plume, 1993)
Breaking Free from Compulsive Eating (Plume, 1993)

MONA LISA SCHULZ, M.D.,Ph.D.
Awakening Intuition: Using Your Mind-Body Network for Insight and Healing (Harmony, 1998)

ANDREW WEIL, M.D.
8 Weeks to Optimum Health (Knopf, 1997)
Spontaneous Healing (Knopf, 1995)
Natural Health, Natural Medicine (Houghton Mifflin, 1995)

DAVID WHYTE
The Heart Aroused: Poetry and Preservation of the Soul in Corporate America (Doubleday, 1996)
House of Belonging (Many Rivers Press, 1996)

Other Books

The Alternative Advisor: The Complete Guide to Natural Therapies and Alternative Treatments by the editors of Time-Life Books (Time-Life Books, 1997)

Alternative Healing: The Complete A–Z Guide to More Than 150 Different Alternative Therapies (revised edition) by Mark Kastner and Hugh Burroughs (Owl, 1996). This wide-ranging volume, with short profiles of 156 modalities from acupuncture to zero balancing, is an excellent source of information on lesser-known therapies.

Bodywork: What Type of Massage to Get—And How to Make the Most of It by Thomas Claire (Morrow, 1995). An encyclopedic guide to the benefits of many body-work practices, including the Alexander technique, aromatherapy massage, reflexology, Rolfing, shiatsu, and Swedish massage.

The Complete Book of Ayurvedic Home Remedies by Vasant Lad (Harmony, 1998). An encyclopedia for self-healing based on ancient Indian principles.

The Complete German Commission E Monographs: Therapeutic Guide to Herbal Medicines translated and edited by the American Botanical Council (ABC, 1998). Originally published by Commission E, the German government's expert committee on herbal remedies, this reference book contains translated monographs on more than 300 herbs, along with information on approved uses, side effects, dosages, and other therapeutic information.

Directory of Schools for Alternative and Complementary Health Care edited by Karen Rappaport (Oryx Press, 1998). A listing of nearly 700 schools for people seeking professional training in alternative health care modalities.

Dr. Fulford's Touch of Life: The Healing Power of the Natural Life Force by Robert C. Fulford, with Gene Stone (Pocket Books, 1996) The well-known osteopath shares his advice for vitality and good health.

Dr. Pitcairn's Complete Guide to Natural Health for Dogs and Cats (revised edition) by Richard H. Pitcairn and Susan Hubble Pitcairn (Rodale, 1995). This comprehensive work includes easy-to-make recipes for healthy pet food and provides information on homeopathic, herbal, and other natural remedies for animal diseases.

Encyclopedia of Natural Medicine by Michael T. Murray and Joseph Pizzorno (Prima, 1991). This classic compendium by two naturopathic physicians discusses the use of herbs, vitamins, minerals, diet, and other treatments for more than 70 conditions and diseases.

Everyday Enlightenment: The Twelve Gateways to Personal Growth by Dan Millman (Warner, 1998). Teachings and exercises for achieving mental and physical well-being by the author of *The Way of the Peaceful Warrior.*

The Five Elements of Self-Healing: Using Chinese Medicine for Maximum Immunity, Wellness, and Health by Jason Elias and Katherine Ketcham (Harmony, 1998). An introduction to the five fundamental elements of Chinese medicine—wood, fire, earth, metal, and water—and guidance on how to achieve mind/body health by keeping them in balance.

Foods That Fight Pain: Revolutionary New Strategies for Maximum Pain Relief by Neal Barnard, M.D. (Harmony, 1998). The author of *Eat Right, Live Longer* tells how to soothe everyday ailments and chronic pain by using common foods, supplements, and herbs.

Food—Your Miracle Medicine by Jean Carper (HarperCollins, 1994). A well-researched and highly readable book on the power of food to prevent or relieve minor ailments, as well as to ward off major killers, including heart disease and cancer.

The Green Pharmacy by James A. Duke (Rodale, 1997). One of the world's leading authorities on medicinal plants describes a variety of healing herbs and rates their effectiveness in treating more than 120 diseases and conditions in this reader-friendly guide.

Herbal Home Remedy Book: Simple Recipes for Tinctures, Teas, Salves, Tonics, and Syrups by Joyce A. Wardwell (Storey Publishing, 1998). Guidance on how to use 25 common plants, including weeds, to relieve everything from allergies to warts.

Herbs of Choice: The Therapeutic Use of Phytomedicinals (Pharmaceutical Products, 1994) and *The Honest Herbal: A Sensible Guide to the Use of Herbs and Related Remedies* (Pharmaceutical Products, 1993) by Varro E. Tyler. A recognized authority on herbs and their uses provides comprehensive information on commonly used herbal medicines. Both books contain scientific references.

The HIV Wellness Sourcebook: An East-West Guide to Living Well with HIV/AIDS and Related Conditions by Misha Ruth Cohen with Kalia Doner (Owl, 1998). A treatment program based on Chinese medicine by an acupuncturist and doctor of Oriental medicine.

The Holistic Pediatrician by Kathi J. Kemper, M.D. (HarperCollins, 1996). This book offers both conventional and complementary approaches to the 25 most common childhood ailments, including bed-wetting, diaper rash, and ear infections.

The Illustrated Encyclopedia of Healing Remedies by C. Norman Shealy, M.D. (Element, 1998). More than 1,000 natural remedies for common ailments and conditions by the renowned neurosurgeon and founder of the American Holistic Medical Association.

Jade Remedies: A Chinese Herbal Reference for the West, Volumes 1 and 2 by Peter Holmes (Snow Lotus Press, 1997). A vast resource for the Western practitioner of Chinese medicine.

Lorna Sass' Short-Cut Vegetarian: Great Taste in No Time by Lorna J. Sass (Quill/Morrow, 1997). One of America's foremost vegetarian chefs shares more than 100 quick and delicious vegan recipes.

Manifesto for a New Medicine: Your Guide to Healing Partnerships and the Wise Use of Alternative Therapies by James S. Gordon, M.D. (Perseus Press, 1996). A leading advisor to the NIH's National Center for Complementary and Alternative Medicine discusses how to combine the best of orthodox and alternative medicine.

Mind/Body Medicine: How to Use Your Mind for Better Health edited by Daniel Goleman and Joel Gurin (Consumer Reports Books, 1995). A consumer-oriented collection of articles by leading researchers on such mind/body techniques as biofeedback, exercise, hypnosis, imagery, and meditation.

The MindBody Prescription: Healing the Body, Healing the Pain by John E. Sarno, M.D. (Warner, 1998). A well-known back doctor details the benefits of a mind/body approach to easing chronic pain.

Miracles of Mind: Exploring Nonlocal Consciousness and Spiritual Healing by Russell Targ and Jane Katra (New World Library, 1998). An exploration of the mind's ability to influence one's capacity to heal.

Natural Alternatives to Over-the-Counter and Prescription Drugs by Michael T. Murray (Morrow, 1994). A naturopathic physician describes alternatives to more than 200 prescription drugs, plus alternatives to over-the-counter medications for the common cold, heartburn, and many other ailments.

Nutrients A to Z: A User's Guide to Foods, Herbs, Vitamins, Minerals, and Supplements by Michael Sharon (Trafalgar Square, 1998). An easy-to-use reference that covers daily dosages and health benefits.

Open Body: Creating Your Own Yoga by Todd Walton with drawings by Vance Lawry (Avon, 1998). A creative approach to basic yoga principles that can enhance flexibility, decrease pain, increase strength, and foster a positive mind/body connection.

The PDR For Herbal Medicines (Medical Economics, 1998). An authoritative guide from the publishers of *The Physician's Desk Reference* that combines the work of Germany's Commission E with the expertise of world-renowned herbal medicine expert Joerg Gruenwald to provide information on more than 600 herbal remedies.

The People's Medical Society's Men's Health and Wellness Encyclopedia by Charles B. Inlander and the staff of the People's Medical Society (Macmillan, 1998). An accessible resource for men by the president of the nonprofit health advocacy organization.

Successful Aging by John W. Rowe, M.D., and Robert L. Kahn (Pantheon, 1998). Evidence from a MacArthur Foundation study validating the benefits of mind/body medicine.

The UC Berkeley Wellness Self-Care Handbook: The Everyday Guide to Prevention & Home Remedies by John Edward Swartzberg, M.D., and Sheldon Margen, M.D. (Rebus, 1998). Practical advice on disease prevention and treatment from the publishers of the *UC Berkeley Wellness Letter.*

Why People Don't Heal and How They Can by Caroline Myss (Three Rivers Press, 1997). The famed medical intuitive discusses the five myths of healing and teaches new methods of dealing with the challenges presented by the body's seven different energy centers.

PROFESSIONAL ASSOCIATIONS

Acupressure. American Oriental Bodywork Therapy Association, *Laurel Oak Corporate Center, Suite 408, 1010 Haddonfield-Berlin Rd., Voorhees NJ 08043; (609) 782-1616; http://www.healthy.net/aobta.*

Acupuncture/Oriental Medicine. American Academy of Medical Acupuncture, *5820 Wilshire Blvd., Suite 500, Los Angeles CA 90036; (800) 521-2262.* American Association of Oriental Medicine, *433 Front St., Catasauqua PA 18032; (610) 266-1433; http://www.aaom.org.*

Alexander Technique. Alexander Technique International, *1692 Massachusetts Ave., Cambridge MA 02138; (617) 497-2242; http://www.ati-net.com.* North American Society of Teachers of the Alexander Technique, *(800) 473-0620.*

Aromatherapy. National Association for Holistic Aromatherapy, *219 Carl St., San Francisco CA 94117-3804; (415) 564-6785.*

Ayurvedic/Indian Medicine. The Ayurvedic Institute, *P.O. Box 23445, Albuquerque NM 87192-1445; (505) 291-9698.*

Biofeedback. Biofeedback Certification Institute of America, *10200 West 44th Ave., Suite 304, Wheat Ridge CO 80033-2840; (303) 420-2902.*

Bodywork. Associated Bodywork & Massage Professionals, *28677 Buffalo Park Rd., Evergreen CO 80439-7347; (800) 458-2267; http://www.abmp.com.* American Oriental Bodywork Therapy Association, *1010 Haddonfield-Berlin Rd., Suite 408, Voorhees NJ 08043; (609) 782-1616.*

Chiropractic. American Chiropractic Association, *1701 Clarendon Blvd., Arlington VA 22209; (703) 276-8800; http://www.amerchiro.org.* International Chiropractors Association, *1110 North Glebe Rd., Suite 1000, Arlington VA 22201; (800) 423-4690; http://www.chiropractic.org.*

Diet. American Dietetic Association, *216 West Jackson Blvd., Chicago IL 60606; (312) 899-0040; http://www.eatright.org.*

Energy Medicine. International Society for the Study of Subtle Energies and Energy Medicine, *356 Goldco Circle, Golden CO 80403; (303) 425-4625; http://www.nekesc.org/~issseem.*

Environmental Medicine. American Academy of Environmental Medicine, *10 Randolph St., New Hope PA 18938; (215) 862-4544; http://www.aaem.com.*

Feldenkrais Method. The Feldenkrais Guild, *P.O. Box 489, Albany OR 97321; (541) 926-0981 or (800) 775-2118; http://www.feldenkrais.com.*

Flower Essences. Flower Essence Society, P.O. Box 1769, Nevada City CA 95959; (530) 265-9163; http://www.floweressence.com.

Herbs. The American Botanical Council, 6200 Manor Rd., Austin TX 78723; (512) 926-4900; http://www.herbalgram.org. The Herb Research Foundation, 1007 Pearl St., Suite 200, Boulder CO 80302; (303) 449-2265; http://www.herbs.org. American Herbalist Guild, P.O. Box 70, Roosevelt UT 84066; http://www.healthy.net/herbalists/index.html.

Homeopathy. American Association of Homeopathic Pharmacists, 1441 West Smith Rd., Ferndale WA 98248; (800) 478-0421. National Center for Homeopathy, 801 North Fairfax St., Suite 306, Alexandria VA 22314; (703) 548-7790; http://www.homeopathic.org.

Hypnosis. American Board of Hypnotherapy, 16842 Von Karman Ave., Suite 475, Irvine CA 92606; (800) 872-9996; http://www.hypnosis.com. American Society of Clinical Hypnosis, 33 West Grand Ave., Suite 402, Chicago IL 60610, (312) 645-9810; http://www.asch.net. National Guild of Hypnotists, P.O. Box 308, Merrimack NH 03054; (603) 429-9438; ngh@ngh.net. International Medical and Dental Hypnotherapy Association, 4110 Edgeland, Suite 800, Royal Oak MI 48073; (248) 549-5594.

Imagery. Academy for Guided Imagery, PO Box 2070, Mill Valley CA 94942; (800) 726-2070.

Massage. American Massage Therapy Association, 820 Davis St., Suite 100, Evanston IL 60201-4444; (847) 864-0123. International Massage Association, 3000 Connecticut Ave. N.W., Suite 308, Washington DC 20008; (202) 387-6555; http://www.imagroup.com. Associated Bodywork & Massage Professionals, 28677 Buffalo Park Rd., Evergreen CO 80439-7347; (800) 458-2267; http://www.abmp.com.

Medicine, Holistic. American Holistic Medical Association, 6728 Old McLean Village Dr., McLean VA 22101; http://www.holisticmedicine.org. The Mind/Body Medical Institute, Beth Israel Deaconess Hospital, Division of Behavioral Medicine, 100 Francis St., Suite 1A, Boston MA 02215; (617) 632-9525.

Midwifery. American College of Nurse-Midwives, 818 Connecticut Ave. N.W., Suite 900, Washington DC 20006; (202) 728-9860; http://www.acnm.org.

Music Therapy. American Music Therapy Association, 8455 Colesville Rd., Suite 1000, Silver Spring MD 20910; (301) 589-3300; http://www.musictherapy.org.

Naturopathy. American Association of Naturopathic Physicians, 601 Valley St., Suite 105, Seattle WA 98109; (206) 298-0125. American Naturopathic

Medical Association, P.O. Box 96273, Las Vegas NV 89193; (702) 897-7053; http://www.anma.com. Bastyr University College of Naturopathic Medicine, 14500 Juanita Dr. N.E., Kenmore WA 98028-4966; (425) 823-1300; http://www.bastyr.edu. Homeopathic Academy of Naturopathic Physicians, 12132 S.E. Foster Place, Portland OR 97266; (503) 761-3298.

Nursing, Holistic. American Holistic Nurses' Association, P.O. Box 2130, Flagstaff AZ 86003-2130; (800) 278-2462; http://www.ahna.org.

Osteopathy. American Osteopathic Association, 142 East Ontario St., Chicago IL 60611; (800) 621-1773; http://www.aoa-net.org.

Polarity Therapy. American Polarity Therapy Association, 2888 Bluff St., Suite 149, Boulder CO 80301; (800) 359-5620; http://www.polaritytherapy.org.

Reflexology. International Institute of Reflexology, P.O. Box 12642, St. Petersburg FL 33733-2642; (813) 343-4811.

Reiki. The Reiki Alliance, P.O. Box 41, Cataldo ID 83810; (208) 682-3535.

Rolfing. The Rolf Institute, 205 Canyon Blvd., Boulder CO 80302; (303) 449-5903.

Rosen Method. Rosen Method Professional Association, referrals only, (800) 893-2622.

Rubenfeld Synergy Method. Rubenfeld Synergy Center, 115 Waverly Place, New York NY 10011; (800)747-6897; http://www.members.aol.com/rubenfeld/synergy/index.html.

Social Work. National Association of Social Workers, 750 First St. S.E., Suite 700, Washington DC; 20002; (202) 408-8600.

Therapeutic Touch. Nurse Healers–Professional Associates International, 1211 Locust St., Philadelphia PA 19107; (215) 545-8079; http://www.therapeutic-touch.org.

Trager. The Trager Institute, 21 Locust Ave., Mill Valley CA 94941; (415) 388-2688.

Veterinary Medicine, Holistic. American Holistic Veterinary Medical Association, 2214 Old Emmorton Rd., Bel Air MD 21015; (410) 569-0795; http://www.altvetmed.com.

Yoga. International Association of Yoga Therapists, 20 Sunnyside Ave., Suite A-243, Mill Valley, CA 94941; (415) 332-2478. B.K.S. Iyengar Yoga National Association of the United States, (800) 889-YOGA.

WHAT DO THOSE INITIALS MEAN?

ABMP Associated Bodywork & Massage Professionals. Members have met educational and state (if applicable) requirements and agree to adhere to a code of professional ethics.

ACSW Academy of Certified Social Workers. Members have passed an exam given by the National Association of Social Workers. Prerequisites include a master's degree in social work (see MSW) and two years of full-time (or 3,000 hours of part-time) post-master's social work experience and supervision.

AMTA American Massage Therapy Association. Members have graduated from an AMTA-accredited or AMTA-approved school; received licensing from an AMTA-approved state, city, or province; or passed the national certification exam administered by the National Certification Board for Therapeutic Massage and Bodywork.

AOBTA American Oriental Bodywork Therapy Association. Professional members have completed at least 500 hours of training in acupressure, shiatsu, and other oriental bodywork therapies. The organization represents certified practitioners.

ARNP Advanced Registered Nurse Practitioner (see NP/ARNP).

BSN Bachelor of Science in Nursing.

CAR Certified Advanced Rolfer. To qualify, an individual must be a certified rolfer for three years and earn 18 continuing education credits through the Rolf Institute.

CCH Certificate in Classical Homeopathy. To qualify, a person must be trained by a recognized program and pass a licensing exam by the Council for Homeopathic Certification of the American Association of Naturopathic Physicians.

CHT Certified Hypnotherapist. Organizations that certify hypnotherapists include the American Board of Hypnotherapy, the International Medical and Dental Hypnotherapy Association, and the American Society of Clinical Hypnosis. Requirements vary.

CISW Certified Independent Social Worker (state certification).

CM Certified Midwife. To qualify, a person must have a background in a health field other than nursing, graduate from an accredited midwifery education program, and pass an exam given by the American College of Nurse-Midwives Certification Council.

CMP/CMT Certified Massage Practitioner/Certified Massage Therapist. These individuals have received a certificate of completion from a school of massage therapy.

CNM Certified Nurse-Midwife. Requires the earning of an RN degree, completion of an accredited graduate-level nurse-midwifery education program, and passage of an exam given by the American College of Nurse-Midwives Certification Council.

CR Certified Rolfer or Certified Reflexologist. Certified Rolfers must have 15 weeks of training at the Rolf Institute. Certified reflexologists pass an exam given by the International Institute of Reflexology.

CSW Certified Social Worker.

CTP Certified Trager Practitioner. Requires the completion of the Trager Institute's professional certification program.

DC Doctor of Chiropractic. Requires four years of training at an accredited chiropractic college. Chiropractors take both national and state board exams and are licensed to practice by state.

DHANP Naturopaths who pass the certification exam given by the Homeopathic Academy of Naturopathic Physicians use these initials.

DHt Awarded by the American Board of Homeotherapeutics, this diploma is only open to licensed medical doctors and doctors of osteopathy.

DiplAc Diplomate in Acupuncture. Indicates that the acupuncturist met the certification requirements of the National Commission for the Certification of Acupuncturists.

DNBHE Diplomate of the National Board of Homeopathic Examiners. Open only to health practitioners (chiropractors, dentists, registered nurses, and others) who are state-licensed to write prescriptions and who pass a comprehensive exam.

DO Doctor of Osteopathy. To become an osteopathic physician, a person must complete four years of training at a college of osteopathic medicine. There are currently 16 such colleges accredited by the American Osteopathy Association.

DVM Doctor of Veterinary Medicine.

GCFP Guild-Certified Feldenkrais Practitioner. Requires the completion of a professional training program accredited by the Feldenkrais Guild.

LAc, LicAc Licensed Acupuncturist. Indicates state licensure or a diploma from a European school.

LCSW Licensed Clinical Social Worker or Licensed Certified Social Worker.

LD Licensed Dietitian.

LMP/LMT Licensed Massage Practitioner/Licensed Massage Therapist. Some states license bodyworkers as "massage practitioners," while other states license them as "massage therapists."

LPN Licensed Practical Nurse. Indicates the completion of a 12- to 14-month post-high-school educational course on basic nursing care. LPNs also must pass a licensing exam.

MAc Master of Acupuncture. Graduate of an MAc education program, accredited by the National Accreditation Commission for Schools and Colleges of Acupuncture and Oriental Medicine.

MFCC Marriage, Family, and Child Counselor. State licensure in California requires one of six relevant master's degrees and 3,000 hours of clinical experience.

MOM Master of Oriental Medicine. Graduate of an MOM education program accredited by the National Accreditation Commission for Schools and Colleges of Acupuncture and Oriental Medicine.

MPH Master of Public Health.

MSN Master of Science in Nursing.

MSW Master of Social Work.

NASTAT North American Society of Teachers of the Alexander Technique. Membership requires 1,600 hours of training over a three-year period at a NASTAT-certified school.

ND Doctor of Naturopathy. Naturopaths are currently licensed in 11 states: Alaska, Arizona, Connecticut, Hawaii, Maine, Montana, New Hampshire, Oregon, Utah, Vermont, and Washington. NDs are required to graduate from a school accredited by the Council on Naturopathic Medical Education or an equivalent foreign school.

NMD Doctor of Naturopathic Medicine. In Arizona, licensed naturopathic physicians may use the ND (see above) or NMD license. The requirements for licensure are the same.

NP/ARNP Nurse Practitioner/Advanced Registered Nurse Practitioner. A registered nurse (RN) who has completed a nurse practitioner education program—usually a master's degree program—in addition to the two to four years of nursing education required of RNs. At least 36 states require nurse practitioners to be nationally certified by the American Nurses Association or by a specialty nursing organization.

OMD/DOM Oriental Medical Doctor/Doctor of Oriental Medicine. These titles generally indicate some additional training beyond state licensure to practice acupuncture and Chinese traditional medicine. These titles may be used by doctors who are licensed in China but not in the United States, or by U.S. practitioners who complete OMD or DOM degree programs outside the United States.

PA Physician Assistant. Graduate of an accredited physician assistant or surgeon assistant educational program (usually two years in length).

PA-C Physician Assistant–Certified. Requires the passage of an exam administered by the National Commission on Certification of Physician Assistants.

PT Physical Therapist. To qualify for this state license, therapists must complete an educational program accredited by the Commission on Accreditation in Physical Therapy Education.

RAc Registered Acupuncturist. Indicates state registration, which may or may not include a review of qualifications.

RD Registered Dietitian. Requires a minimum of four years of education and training in dietetics or a related field at a university accredited by the American Dietetic Association and the passage of an exam given by the Commission on Dietetic Registration. RDs must fulfill continuing educational requirements to maintain their title.

RM Reiki Master. The traditional criteria include at least three years as a Reiki practitioner and at least one year as an apprentice to a Reiki Master. RMs belong to the Reiki Alliance, whose members uphold professional standards. The organization does not offer certification.

RMT Registered Massage Therapist. The American Massage Therapy Association (see AMTA) no longer grants this title, which certifies advanced training in massage therapy. However, people who previously qualified for the title may continue to use it.

RN Registered Nurse. Requires the graduation from a state-approved school of nursing (two to four years in length) and passage of a state licensing exam.

RP Registered Polarity Practitioner. Requires 615 hours of training in polarity therapy; recognized by the American Polarity Therapy Association.

WELLNESS ON THE WORLD WIDE WEB

Alternative Medicine Digest This site features articles on many aspects of alternative care, from natural remedies to the politics of medicine. *http://www.alternativemedicine.com*

Ask Dr. Weil Andrew Weil's site includes the popular "Ask Dr. Weil" daily Q & A column, newsgroups, excerpts from his book *Natural Health, Natural Medicine,* and links to other resources. The site also features a referral directory of herbalists and other practitioners of alternative medicine. *http://www.drweil.com*

BodyAtlas BodyAtlas offers medical, health, and wellness information from conventional and alternative medicine experts. *http://www.bodywise.net*

CyberDiet If you've got questions about nutrition, this site can help you answer them. Find out your daily calorie and nutrient requirements, then plan your menu, shopping lists, and recipes accordingly. *http://www.cyberdiet.com*

FeMiNa: Health and Wellness is one of the largest resources on the Internet for women's issues. The "Ask a Woman Doctor" link connects you to women physicians who can answer your health questions online, and other links provide contact information for women's health clinics, midwives, massage therapists, and other women's health care providers throughout North America. *http://www.femina.cybergrrl.com/femina/HealthandWellness*

GriefNet For anyone who has lost a loved one, this site serves as both a resource and a source of comfort. *http://www.griefnet.org*

HealthGate A prime online source for health, wellness, and biomedical information, HealthGate contains extensive material on both alternative and conventional medicine. For registered users (registration is free), the "Patient Education" page connects you to guides to illnesses, medical tests, surgeries, and prescription and over-the-counter drugs. *http://www.healthgate.com*

HealthWorld Online Combining elements of allopathic and alternative medicine, this site offers information on wellness, self-care, fitness, nutrition, and a wide array of health conditions. An online professional referral network is also provided. *http://www.healthy.net*

HealthWWWeb Integrative medicine, natural health, and alternative therapies are the bill of fare at this site. *http://www.health wwweb.com*

Healthy Ideas This excellent, encyclopedic site from *Prevention* magazine covers such topics as weight loss, fitness, healthy cooking, family health, and natural living. *http://www.prevention.com*

HerbNet If you are an herbalist, a chef, or a gardener, you will delight in this online resource, which features detailed information on the medical, culinary, and ritual uses of herbs. *http://www.herbnet.com*

Homeopathy Home Page. The stated goal of this site is to provide links to every homeopathy resource available. While it's impossible to say whether it actually achieves this, it probably comes close. *http://www.homeopathyhome.com*

Institute for Traditional Medicine. The site of the Portland, Oregon–based Institute for Traditional Medicine focuses on Chinese herbal medicine, but it provides much information on the ayurvedic, Tibetan, Native American, and Thai medical traditions as well. *http://www.europa.com/~itm*

The International Center for Reiki Training This site is designed primarily for Reiki students and practitioners, but it also covers a lot of basic information on the history, principles, and uses of this form of energy healing. *http://www.reiki.org*

Mayo Health O@sis The Mayo Clinic sponsors this comprehensive site, which spans topics ranging from allergies to Alzheimer's disease. *http://www.mayohealth.org*

Mental Health Net This guide to mental health, psychology, and psychiatry lists more than 7,000 resources and features the latest mental health news. *http://www.cmhc.com*

NCCAM The National Institutes of Health's National Center for Complementary and Alternative Medicine (formerly the Office of Alternative Medicine). The site includes information on research grants and the NCCAM Clearinghouse, which disseminates information on complementary and alternative medicine to practitioners and the public. *http://altmed.od.nih.gov/nccam*

OncoLink The University of Pennsylvania Cancer Center Resource. This award-winning site includes pages on cancer causes, screening and prevention, clinical trials of new treatments, financial issues for patients, and coping with grief and loss. *http://www.oncolink.org*

PubMed This search service allows you to access the 9,000,000 citations in MedLine and other medical databases free of charge. *http://www.ncbi.nlm.nih.gov/PubMed*

Sapient Health Network Developed for people with chronic and serious illnesses, this interactive health service provides a wealth of useful information and support. *http://www.shn.net/corp.html*

Southwest School of Botanical Medicine Michael Moore, director of the Southwest School of Botanical Medicine in Bisbee, Arizona, maintains what is easily the most comprehensive resource online for information on medicinal plants. *http://chili.rt66.com/hrbmoore/HOMEPAGE/HomePage.html*

Thrive This online service devoted to healthy living is a useful and spirited resource for information on health, fitness, food, and sexuality. *http://www.thriveonline.com*

Wellness Web Dubbing itself "The Patient's Network," this site covers aspects of both conventional and alternative medicine, touching on everything from cancer to cholesterol to quitting smoking. *http://www.wellweb.com*

Yahoo!'s Alternative Medicine This page offers links to numerous indices, organizations, and practitioners of various alternative health modalities, as well as short reviews of several dozen of the best sites. Yahoo!'s simple format allows you to browse topic by topic or to conduct keyword searches on subjects ranging from acupuncture to zinc.
http://www.yahoo.com/health/alternative_medicine

FOR MORE INFORMATION

Adventure Game Theater

This nonprofit company specializes in creating community through play, ritual, and theater. Adventure Game Theater provides workshops for organizations, corporations, and schools and also offers summer camps for teens.

Adventure Game Theater
P.O. Box 416
Lee MA 01238
(888) 792-PLAY
http://www.agt.org

Body & Soul

The leading national conference series on mind/body healing, spirituality, creativity, and social transformation. For information, call (800) 944-1001

Center for Mindfulness/Stress Reduction Clinic

The first hospital-based stress reduction clinic in the country, founded by Jon Kabat-Zinn.

Center for Mindfulness/Stress Reduction Clinic
University of Massachusetts Medical Center
55 Lake Ave. North
Worcester MA 01655-0267.

Center for Science in the Public Interest

This nutrition advocacy group is one of the nation's best sources of information about the quality of food.

Center for Science in the Public Interest
1875 Connecticut Ave. N.W., Suite 300
Washington DC 20009
(202) 332-9110
http://www.cspinet.org

Commonweal Cancer Help Program

Founded by Michael Lerner, this program offers weeklong retreats for cancer patients and their loved ones.

Commonweal Cancer Help Program
P.O. Box 316
Bolinas CA 94924
(415) 868-0970
http://www.commonwealhealth.org

Dr. Andrew Weil's Self Healing
A monthly newsletter on natural health for body and mind from the trusted
integrative medicine expert Andrew Weil, M.D. Bound annual editions from
1996 to the present are also available. For subscription information, call
(800) 523-3296.

Food & Water, Inc.
This organization addresses food safety issues such as food irradiation and
bovine growth hormone use.

Food & Water, Inc.
389 Vermont Route 215
Walden VT 05873
(800) EAT-SAFE

The Inner Voyage
An annual transformational travel event featuring visionary authors, experien-
tial workshop leaders, and experts on intuition, astrology, dreamwork, yoga,
meditation, and more. For information, call (800) 546-7871

Mothers & Others for a Livable Planet
This group, cofounded by actress Meryl Streep, concentrates on the use of
agricultural pesticides and other issues of relevance to children's health.

Mothers & Others for a Livable Planet
40 W. 20th St.
New York NY 10011
(888) ECO-INFO
http://www.mothers.org/mothers

Omega Institute
The nation's largest holistic education and retreat center, offering more than
250 workshops, spiritual retreats, conferences, and other activities.

Omega Institute
260 Lake Dr.
Rhinebeck NY 12572
(800) 944-1001
http://www.omega-inst.org

New Age: The Journal for Holistic Living
America's leading magazine on holistic living, alternative health, and spirituality for the past 25 years. *New Age* is published bimonthly, plus three special issues: *Body & Soul: The Annual Guide to Holistic Living, Body & Soul: Guide to Holistic Health,* and *Body & Soul Buyers' Guide.* For subscription information, call (800) 755-1178.

Program in Integrative Medicine
Directed by Andrew Weil, M.D., this is the first program of its kind to train physicians and other health professionals to integrate the best of conventional and alternative medicine.

Program in Integrative Medicine
P.O. Box 245153
Tucson AZ 85724-5153
http://www.ahsc.arizona.edu/integrative_medicine

The Vegetarian Resource Group
This group offers a wealth of information on vegetarian lifestyles, nutrition, and travel, as well as vegetarian recipes.

The Vegetarian Resource Group
P.O. Box 1463
Baltimore MD 21203
(410) 366-VEGE
http://www.vrg.org

GLOSSARY

ACUPRESSURE Based on the principles of acupuncture, this ancient Chinese technique involves the use of finger pressure (rather than needles) at specific points along the body to treat ailments such as tension and stress, aches and pains, menstrual cramps, or arthritis. Acupressure is also used for general preventive health care.

ACUPUNCTURE In acupuncture, fine needles are inserted at specific points to stimulate, disperse, and regulate the flow of *chi*, or vital energy, and to restore a healthy energy balance. Often used in the United States for pain relief, acupuncture is also used to improve well-being and treat acute, chronic, and degenerative conditions in children and adults.

AIKIDO Like other Japanese martial arts, aikido is both a method of self-defense and a spiritual discipline. The goal is to harmonize one's *chi* (vital energy) with that of one's opponent, so that the opponent's strength and weight are used against him or her. Many of the moves are flowing and graceful, similar to those of tai chi.

ALEXANDER TECHNIQUE This mind/body technique was developed by actor F. Matthias Alexander, who created the method after concluding that bad posture was responsible for his own chronic voice loss. Practitioners, using gentle hands-on guidance and verbal instruction, teach simple, efficient ways of moving as a means to improve balance, posture, and coordination and to relieve tension and pain.

ALLOPATHIC MEDICINE Originally coined by homeopathic physician Samuel Hahnemann in the 19th century, the term *allopathic medicine* is derived from Greek roots meaning "other than the disease." Although Hahnemann used the term to describe medical practice that prescribed drugs with no logical relationship to symptoms, the term is used most often today to distinguish it from alternative modalities such as homeopathy, herbal medicine, etc. Also known as conventional medicine.

AMMA THERAPY This system of bodywork therapy uses traditional Asian medical principles for assessing and evaluating imbalances in the energetic system. AMMA therapy aims to restore, promote, and maintain optimum health through the treatment of the physical body, the bio-energy, and the emotions. It is used for a wide range of medical conditions.

ANTHROPOSOPHIC MEDICINE Developed by philosopher and mystic Rudolf Steiner, this medical system takes into account the spiritual and physical components of illness. A treatment regime may include herbal and homeopathic medicines as well as dietary recommendations, art therapy, movement therapy, massage, and specially prepared baths.

ANTIOXIDANT Antioxidants are substances that protect against the oxidation of free radicals, dangerous chemical compounds that promote disease. The vitamins C and E, beta-carotene, and selenium are well-known antioxidants.

APPLIED KINESIOLOGY This system uses muscle-testing procedures in conjunction with standard methods of diagnosis to gain information about a patient's overall state of health. Practitioners analyze muscle function, posture, gait, and other structural factors and inquire about lifestyle factors that may be contributing to a health-related problem. Nutritional supplements, muscle and joint manipulation, and lifestyle modification (including diet and exercise) may then be used as part of a treatment plan. Applied kinesiology is used by healthcare providers who are licensed to diagnose, such as chiropractors, osteopaths, dentists, and medical doctors.

AROMATHERAPY Aromatherapy uses "essential oils" (the volatile oils distilled from plants) to treat emotional disorders such as stress and anxiety as well as a wide range of other ailments. Oils are inhaled, massaged into the skin in diluted form, or placed in baths. Aromatherapy is often used in conjunction with massage therapy, acupuncture, reflexology, herbology, chiropractic, and other holistic treatments.

ASTROLOGY Astrology is the study of the positions of the planets in the solar system and their possible influence on human affairs. Based on this information, a counselor can work with a client to provide individualized insights into emotional, professional, and health matters or into the client's personality.

AYURVEDIC MEDICINE Practiced in India for more than 5,000 years, the ayurvedic tradition holds that illness is a state of imbalance among the body's systems that can be detected through such diagnostic procedures as reading the pulse and observing the tongue. Nutrition counseling, massage, natural medications, meditation, and other modalities are used to address a broad spectrum of ailments, from allergies to AIDS. Maharishi Ayur-Ved is a contemporary interpretation of ayurvedic medicine inspired by Maharishi Mahesh Yogi, the founder of Transcendental Meditation.

BARBARA BRENNAN HEALING SCIENCE Developed by physicist, teacher, and healer Barbara Brennan, this spiritual healing system seeks to reorganize and heal the client's energy field. Using both hands-on techniques and other approaches, the healer works to clear the client's field of unhealthy and blocked energies, charge depleted areas, repair distorted patterns, and balance the entire field. The goal is to promote health and healing on physical, emotional, mental, and spiritual levels.

BIOENERGETICS Bioenergetics holds that repressed emotions and desires affect the body and psyche by creating chronic muscle tension and diminished vitality and energy. Through physical exercises, breathing techniques, verbal psychotherapy, or other forms of emotional-release work, the therapist attempts to loosen this "character armor" and restore natural well-being.

BIOFEEDBACK A technique used especially for stress-related conditions such as asthma, migraines, insomnia, and high blood pressure, biofeedback is a way of monitoring minute metabolic changes in one's own body (e.g., temperature changes, heart rate, and muscle tension) with the aid of sensitive machines. By consciously visualizing, relaxing, or imagining while observing light, sound, or metered feedback, the client learns to make subtle adjustments to move toward a more balanced internal state.

BODY-MIND CENTERING Body-mind centering is a movement-reeducation approach that explores how the body's systems (skeletal, muscular, nervous, etc.) contribute to movement and self-awareness. The approach also emphasizes movement patterns that develop during infancy and childhood. Body-mind centering incorporates guided movement, exercise, imagery, and hands-on work. The approach can be used with infants, children, and adults to resolve movement problems and facilitate the "mind/body dialogue."

BODY-MIND COUNSELING This is a general term for a range of practices that combine bodywork with some form of verbal dialogue. *Counseling* can suggest a less formally systematic approach than does the term *psychotherapy*, and it can also encompass advice about diet or lifestyle issues.

BODY-ORIENTED PSYCHOTHERAPY Body-oriented psychotherapy seeks to enhance the psychotherapeutic process by incorporating a range of massage, bodywork, and movement techniques. Acknowledging the mind/body link, practitioners may use light touch, soft- or deep-tissue manipulation, breathing techniques, movement, exercise, or body-awareness techniques to help address emotional issues.

BODYWORK FOR ABUSE SURVIVORS Massage therapists and bodyworkers in this category work with survivors of sexual abuse to assign new meaning to touch and develop healthy boundaries as part of their recovery process. This work is often done in direct collaboration with a psychotherapist.

BONNIE PRUDDEN MYOTHERAPY Developed by a fitness expert in 1976, this bodywork method is intended to relax muscle spasms, improve circulation, and alleviate pain. The practitioner, using elbows, knuckles, or fingers, applies pressure for several seconds to trigger points—highly irritable spots on muscle tissue that may radiate pain to other areas. Clients also perform specific exercises for the freed muscles.

BREATHWORK Breathwork is a general term for a variety of techniques that use patterned breathing to promote physical, mental, and/or spiritual well-being. Some techniques use the breath in a calm, peaceful way to induce relaxation or manage pain, while others use stronger breathing to stimulate emotions and emotional release.

BREEMA BODYWORK Breema bodywork is an ancient, nondiagnostic health-improvement method that uses a series of gentle, rhythmic movements to release tension and promote health, vitality, and inner harmony. Treatments are designed to create structural, physiological, emotional, and energetic balance in both the practitioner and the recipient. Breema bodywork is done fully clothed, with the recipient lying or sitting on a carpeted floor.

CAREER/LIFE COUNSELING (LIFE COACHING) Practitioners of career/life counseling assist clients in career planning and/or personal planning and decision-making. Holistic counselors often use a "whole person" approach rather than a strictly vocational approach.

CHELATION THERAPY Typically administered in an osteopathic or medical doctor's office, chelation therapy is a series of intravenous injections of the synthetic amino acid EDTA, designed to detoxify the body. Chelation therapy is also often used to treat arteriosclerosis.

CHINESE (ORIENTAL) MEDICINE Oriental medical practitioners are trained to use a variety of ancient and modern therapeutic methods—including acupuncture, herbal medicine, massage, moxibustion (heat therapy), and nutritional and lifestyle counseling—to treat a broad range of both chronic and acute illnesses.

CHI-KUNG (*see QI GONG*)

CHIROPRACTIC The chiropractic system is based on the premise that the spine is literally the backbone of human health. Misalignments of the vertebrae caused by poor posture or trauma result in pressure on the spinal nerve roots, which may lead to diminished function and illness. The chiropractor seeks to analyze and correct these misalignments through spinal manipulation or adjustment.

COENZYME Q-10 ("COQ-10") A natural substance that assists in oxidative metabolism. CoQ-10 in supplement form may benefit heart patients and people with cancer and chronic diseases.

COLON THERAPY Colon therapy involves the cleansing of the large intestine with warm purified water. A single colonic treatment is said to be equivalent to several enemas in removing toxic debris from the colon.

COMPLEMENTARY MEDICINE Treatments or therapies that complement rather than replace conventional medical (allopathic) practice. Such therapies may include herbal medicine, bodywork, mind/body modalities, etc.

CONSCIOUS BODYWORK This form of neuromuscular reprogramming and therapy combines massage techniques with muscle testing in order to help people learn how to use their muscles with greater strength and less effort. Conscious bodywork is used to treat persistent joint and muscle pain and to treat restrictions of movement caused by injury.

CORE ENERGETICS Core energetics is a form of body-oriented psychotherapy that aims to break down the client's defenses in order to reach the "core" level of consciousness, or spiritual self. By using bodywork and counseling techniques and offering spiritual guidance, the practitioner seeks to evoke cathartic reactions that open the way to "core energy," enabling the client to become a more loving, creative, receptive, and vibrant person.

CRANIOSACRAL THERAPY Craniosacral therapy is a manual therapeutic procedure for remedying distortions in the structure and function of the craniosacral mechanism—the brain and spinal cord, the bones of the skull, the sacrum, and interconnected membranes. The therapy is used to treat chronic pain, migraine headaches, TMJ, and a range of other conditions. It is performed by a range of licensed health practitioners.

DANCE/MOVEMENT THERAPIES Dance and/or movement therapy uses expressive movement as a therapeutic tool for both personal expression and psychological or emotional healing. Practitioners work with people with physical disabilities, addiction issues, sexual abuse histories, eating disorders, and other concerns.

DEEP-TISSUE BODYWORK This is a general term for a range of therapies that seek to improve the function of the body's connective tissues and/or muscles. Among the conditions deep-tissue bodywork treats are whiplash, low back and neck pain, and degenerative diseases such as multiple sclerosis.

DHA (DOCOSAHEXAENOIC ACID) An omega-3 essential fatty acid found in salmon, flaxseed, and other food sources as well as in supplement form. Studies suggest that deficiencies in DHA may be associated with cognitive decline in older people.

EAR CANDLING Ear candling (also called ear coning) involves placing the narrow end of a specially designed hollow candle at the entry of the ear canal, while the opposite end is lit. Primarily used for wax buildup and related hearing problems, ear candling is also used for ear infections and sinus infections.

ECHINACEA An immune-enhancing herb derived from the ornamental purple coneflower, commonly used to stave off cold or flu symptoms. German research has confirmed echinacea's antiviral and immune-enhancing properties.

ENERGY FIELD WORK Practitioners of this range of therapies look for weaknesses in the energy field in and around the client's body and seek to restore its proper circulation and balance. Energy channeled through the practitioner is directed to strengthen the body's natural defenses and help the client's physical, mental, emotional, and/or spiritual state. Sessions may or may not involve the physical laying-on of hands.

EXPRESSIVE THERAPIES Expressive therapies use the arts to promote physical health, mental health, and/or personal growth. Examples of expressive therapies include art therapy, dance therapy, drama therapy, music therapy, poetry therapy, and psychodrama.

FASTING/NATURAL HYGIENE Natural hygiene is a health system that seeks to remove the causes of disease and encourage the body's self-healing capacity through natural-food diets and therapeutic fasting. Professional natural hygienists are primary care doctors (M.D.s, osteopaths, chiropractors, and naturopaths) who specialize in fasting supervision as a part of natural hygienic care. Natural hygiene is employed for a wide variety of acute and chronic conditions.

FELDENKRAIS METHOD The Feldenkrais method combines movement training, gentle touch, and verbal dialogue to help create freer, more efficient movement. Feldenkrais takes two forms: In individual hands-on sessions ("functional integration"), the practitioner's touch is used to address the student's breathing and body alignment, and in a series of classes of slow, nonaerobic motions ("awareness through movement"), students "relearn" improved ways their bodies can move. The Feldenkrais method is frequently used to treat stress and tension, to prevent recurring injury, and to help athletes and others improve their balance and coordination.

FENG SHUI Feng shui (pronounced "fung shway") is the ancient Chinese practice of configuring home or work environments to promote health, happiness, and prosperity. Feng shui consultants may advise clients to make adjustments in their surroundings—from color selection to furniture placement—in order to promote a healthy flow of *chi*, or vital energy.

FLOWER ESSENCES Popularized in the 1930s by Edward Bach, M.D., flower essences are intended to alleviate negative emotional states that may contribute to illness or hinder personal growth. Drops of a solution infused with the captured "essence" of a flower are placed under the tongue or in a beverage. The practitioner helps the client choose appropriate essences, focusing on the client's emotional state rather than on a particular physical condition.

FOCUSING This self-help tool is based on the premise that information about one's life issues can be accessed through a so-called "felt sense" in the body. This skill can be used either alone or in partnership with someone else for resolving day-to-day issues (such as decision-making), negotiating profound changes (such as recovery from abuse), and fostering spiritual development.

GESTALT THERAPY This psychotherapy aims to help the client achieve wholeness (*gestalt* is the German word for "whole") by becoming fully aware of his or her feelings, perceptions, and behavior. The emphasis is on the "here and now" of immediate experience rather than on the past. Gestalt therapy is often conducted in group settings, such as weekend workshops.

GINKGO BILOBA An extract derived from the fan-shaped leaves of the ginkgo tree that improves circulation, inhibits blood clotting, and acts as an antioxidant. Research suggests that ginkgo biloba extract may help improve cognitive function in Alzheimer's patients.

GUIDED IMAGERY Guided imagery involves using mental images to promote physical healing or changes in attitudes or behavior. Practitioners may lead clients through visualization exercises or offer instruction in using imagery as a self-help tool. Guided imagery is often used to alleviate stress and to treat stress-related conditions such as insomnia and high blood pressure. It is also used by people with cancer, AIDS, chronic fatigue syndrome, and other disorders in order to boost the immune system.

GYROTONICS Gyrotonics (also referred to as gyrotonics expansion system or GXS) is an exercise system emphasizing circular motions similar to those used in swimming, tai chi, and yoga. The low-impact exercises are performed on specially designed exercise equipment, and the movements are accompanied by specific breathing patterns. Gyrotonics is used by dancers, athletes, and others to increase strength, flexibility, coordination, and balance. It is also used as a form of physical therapy.

HEALING TOUCH Healing touch is practiced by registered nurses and others to accelerate wound healing, relieve pain, promote relaxation, prevent illness, or ease the dying process. The practitioner uses light touch or works with his or her hands near the client's body in an effort to restore balance to the client's energy system.

HELLERWORK Developed by former aerospace engineer (and one-time Rolf Institute president) Joseph Heller, this technique combines deep-tissue muscle therapy and movement reeducation with dialogue about the emotional issues that may underlie a physical posture. Participants go through 11 60- to 90-minute sessions. Stressing the mind/body connection, Hellerwork is used to treat chronic pain or to help "well" people learn to live more comfortably in their bodies.

HERBALISM An ancient form of healing still widely used in much of the world, herbalism uses natural plants or plant-based substances to treat a range of illnesses and to enhance the functioning of the body's systems. Though herbalism is not a licensed professional modality in the United States, herbs are "prescribed" by a range of practitioners, from holistic M.D.s to acupuncturists and naturopathic physicians.

HOLISTIC DENTISTRY Holistic dentists are licensed dentists who bring an interdisciplinary approach to their practice, often incorporating such methods as homeopathy, nutrition, and acupuncture into their treatment plans. Most holistic dentists emphasize wellness and preventive care and avoid silver-mercury fillings, favoring fillings that do not contain mercury instead.

HOLISTIC MEDICINE Holistic medicine is a broadly descriptive term for a healing philosophy that views a patient as a whole person, not as just a disease or a collection of symptoms. In the course of treatment, holistic medical practitioners may address a client's emotional and spiritual dimensions as well as the nutritional, environmental, and lifestyle factors that may contribute to an illness. Many holistic medical practitioners combine conventional forms of treatment (such as medication and surgery) with natural or alternative treatments.

HOLOTROPIC BREATHWORK Holotropic (which means "moving toward wholeness") breathwork combines accelerated breathing and evocative music played to induce a nonordinary state of consciousness. Holotropic breathwork loosens psychological defenses and leads to a release of unconscious material, which is facilitated by focused bodywork that involves massage and pressure at areas of accumulated tension in the body. Holotropic breathwork can free blocked energies, resulting in the spontaneous healing of old, forgotten psychological traumas.

HOMEOPATHY Homeopathy is a medical system that uses infinitesimal doses of natural substances—called remedies—to stimulate a person's immune and defense system. A remedy is individually chosen for a sick person based on its capacity to cause, if given in overdose, physical and psychological symptoms similar to those the patient is experiencing. Common conditions homeopathy addresses are infant and childhood diseases, infections, fatigue, allergies, and chronic illnesses such as arthritis and asthma.

HYPNOTHERAPY The term hypnotherapy refers to a range of techniques that allow practitioners to bypass the conscious mind and access the subconscious, where suppressed memories, repressed emotions, and forgotten events may remain recorded. Hypnosis may facilitate behavioral, emotional, or attitudinal change. Often used to help people lose weight or stop smoking, it is also used to treat phobias and stress and as an adjunct in the treatment of illnesses.

INTEGRATIVE MEDICINE Integrative medicine is based on a physician-patient partnership within which conventional and alternative modalities are used to stimulate the body's natural healing potential. This approach to healing neither rejects conventional medicine nor uncritically accepts alternative practices.

INTUITIVE ARTS A general term for various methods of divination, including numerology, psychic reading, and tarot reading. Individuals may consult practitioners to seek information about the future or insights into personal concerns or the personality. Among the modalities: Numerology emphasizes the significance of numbers derived from the spelling of names, birth dates, and other significant references; psychics may claim various abilities, from finding lost objects and persons to communicating with the spirits of the dead; and tarot readers interpret a deck of cards containing archetypal symbols.

IRIDOLOGY Iridology is a diagnostic system based on the premise that every organ has a corresponding location within the iris of the eye that can serve as an indicator of the organ's health or disease. Iridology is used by naturopaths and other practitioners, particularly when a diagnosis achieved through standard methods is unclear.

JIN SHIN DO BODYMIND ACUPRESSURE Developed by a psychotherapist, jin shin do combines acupressure, Taoist yogic breathing methods, and Reichian segmental theory (which addresses how emotional tension affects the physical body), with the goal of releasing physical and emotional tension and "armoring." It aims to promote a pleasant trance state in which the participant can address the emotional factors that may underlie various physical conditions.

JIN SHIN JYUTSU Jin shin jyutsu is an Asian system intended to harmonize the flow of energy through the body. The system holds that tension, fatigue, and illness can trap energy in the body's 26 "safety energy locks." Practitioners use their hands to restore balance and reduce stress. Jin shin jyutsu is not a form of massage, however, as it does not involve the physical manipulation of muscles.

KINESIOLOGY/APPLIED KINESIOLOGY Kinesiology is the study of muscles and their movements. Applied kinesiology is a system that uses muscle testing procedures, in conjunction with standard methods of diagnosis, to gain information about a patient's overall state of health. Practitioners analyze muscle function, posture, gait, and other structural factors and inquire about lifestyle factors that may be contributing to a health-related problem. Nutritional supplements, muscle and joint manipulation, and lifestyle modification (including diet and exercise) may then be used as part of a treatment plan. Applied kinesiology is used by healthcare providers who are licensed to diagnose, such as chiropractors, osteopaths, dentists, and medical doctors.

KRIPALU BODYWORK Based on the principles of Kripalu yoga, this bodywork method seeks to promote a deep state of relaxation and help recipients reconnect with the healing wisdom of their bodies. Along with specific massage strokes, Kripalu bodyworkers use verbal and nonverbal means to guide recipients into a meditative state in which physical and mental tension may be accessed and released.

KRIPALU YOGA Kripalu yoga uses classical hatha yoga postures and breathing techniques to help students enter a state of "meditation in motion." Kripalu yoga teachers offer guidance in these yoga techniques and provide an atmosphere in which sensations, thoughts, and emotions can be experienced in safety and relaxation. The principles of Kripalu yoga are the foundations for phoenix rising yoga therapy and Kripalu bodywork.

MACROBIOTICS A low-fat, high-fiber "macrobiotic" diet is based on whole grains, vegetables, sea vegetables, and seeds. A diet of these natural foods, cooked in accordance with macrobiotic principles designed to synchronize one's eating habits with the cycles of nature, is used to promote health and minimize disease. Macrobiotic cookbooks can be found at most health food stores.

MAGNET THERAPY Magnet therapy (also known as magnetic field therapy or bio-magnetic therapy) involves the use of magnets, magnetic devices, or magnetic fields to treat a variety of physical and emotional conditions, including circulatory problems, certain forms of arthritis, chronic pain, sleep disorders, and stress. Treatments may be applied by a practitioner or as part of a self-care program.

MASSAGE, INFANT Taught to new parents by trained instructors, infant massage practices are designed to enhance the bonding between parent and baby. As preventive therapy, infant massage can help strengthen and regulate a baby's respiratory, circulatory, and gastrointestinal functions.

MASSAGE, SWEDISH   The most commonly practiced form of massage in Western countries, Swedish massage integrates ancient eastern techniques with modern principles of anatomy and physiology. Practitioners rub, knead, pummel, brush, and tap the muscles. Swedish massage is widely practiced, and practitioners vary greatly in their training, technique, and length of sessions.

MASSAGE THERAPY This is a general term for a range of therapeutic approaches with roots in both eastern and western cultures. It involves the practice of kneading or otherwise manipulating a person's muscles or other soft tissue with the intent of improving a person's well-being or health.

MEDICAL INTUITIVE A health professional who uses intuition to discern a patient's physical condition and emotional health without seeing the patient, on the basis of minimal information, such as name and age.

MEDITATION Meditation is a general term for a wide range of practices that involve training one's attention or awareness so that one's body and mind can be brought into greater harmony. While some meditators may seek a mystical sense of oneness with a higher power or with the universe, others may seek to reduce stress or alleviate stress-related ailments such as anxiety disorders and high blood pressure.

MIDWIFERY/CHILDBIRTH SUPPORT Midwives provide education and support during pregnancy, assist the mother during labor and delivery, and provide follow-up care. Practitioners of childbirth support include childbirth educators, childbirth assistants, and *doulas* (women labor coaches who also provide postpartum home care). In some states, midwives can attend home births or practice in birthing clinics in hospitals. Some midwives are also licensed to provide "well-women" gynecological care, including screening tests and birth control.

MILK THISTLE An herb used to treat liver conditions such as hepatitis and cirrhosis. Research suggests that silymarin, an extract of milk thistle seeds, has a protective and regenerative effect on the liver.

MINDFUL EATING The attempt to bring non-judgmental awareness to the act of eating and to one's relationship with food.

MINDFUL PARENTING The attempt to bring moment to moment non-judgmental awareness into all aspects of one's life as a parent. Mindfulness brought to parenting has the potential to nourish children through the conscious embodied presence of the parents, which nourishes the parents as well. The foundations of mindful parenting are the cultivation and according of sovereignty (seeing and honoring who the child actually is), empathy, and acceptance.

MINDFULNESS Moment to moment non-judgmental awareness. Often spoken of as the heart of Buddhist meditation.

MINDFULNESS MEDITATION The cultivation of mindfulness through moment to moment non-judgmental attention. One can develop and refine mindfulness by cultivating attention to various objects in one's field of awareness, such as the flowing of one's breath, body sensations, sounds, thoughts, feelings, perceptions of all kinds, impulses, and one's relationship to the world. Mindfulness meditation involves an ongoing effort to cultivate attention through the practice of specific methods (formal meditation practice) and through moment to moment awareness of all aspects of daily life (informal meditation practice).

MUSCULAR THERAPY This general term incorporates a range of bodywork methods and practices that have a therapeutic (not simply relaxing) intent. Practitioners stress client education and follow-up. Among the conditions muscular therapy addresses are chronic back pain, headaches, tension, and emotional illnesses.

MUSIC/SOUND THERAPIES These therapies use music and/or sound to help clients attain therapeutic goals, which may be mental, physical, emotional, social, or spiritual in nature.

MYOFASCIAL RELEASE This hands-on technique seeks to free the body from the grip of tight fascia, or connective tissue, thus restoring normal alignment and function and reducing pain. Using their hands, therapists apply mild, sustained pressure in order to gently stretch and soften the fascia. Myofascial release is used to treat neck and back pain, headaches, recurring sports injuries, and scoliosis, among other conditions.

NATUROPATHIC MEDICINE Naturopathic medicine, a primary healthcare system emphasizing the curative power of nature, treats both acute and chronic illnesses in all age groups. Naturopathic physicians work to restore and support the body's own healing ability using a variety of modalities including nutrition, herbal medicine, homeopathic medicine, and oriental medicine.

NEUROLINGUISTIC PROGRAMMING Neurolinguistic programming is a set of techniques whose goal is to alter limiting patterns of thought, behavior, and language. In conversation, practitioners observe the client's language, eye movements, posture, breathing, and gestures in order to detect and then help change unconscious patterns linked to the client's emotional state.

NEUROMUSCULAR THERAPY Neuromuscular therapy emphasizes the role of the brain, spine, and nerves in muscular pain. One goal of the therapy is to relieve tender, congested spots in muscle tissue and compressed nerves that may radiate pain to other areas of the body.

OHASHIATSU Ohashiatsu is a system of physical techniques, exercises, and meditation used to relieve tension and fatigue and to induce a state of harmony and peace. The practitioner first assesses a person's state by feeling the *hara* (the area below the navel). Then, using continuous and flowing movements, the practitioner presses and stretches the body's energy channels, working in unison with the person's breathing.

OMEGA-3 ESSENTIAL FATTY ACIDS Highly unsaturated fats found in certain types of fish, flaxseed, and other food sources. Research has shown that omega-3s lower the risk of heart attack, reduce inflammation, and possibly help protect against cancer.

OPTION METHOD This personal growth method, which uses a question-and-answer dialogue process, seeks to help people identify and unravel their self-defeating and limiting beliefs in order to achieve happiness, well-being, and creative freedom. The method may be used by teachers, psychotherapists, body-workers, and other professionals who deal with their clients' belief systems. It can be used in private sessions, groups, or workshops and as a self-help tool.

ORTHO-BIONOMY Developed by a British osteopath, ortho-bionomy involves the use of noninvasive, gentle touch along with dialogue and instruction in common movements such as walking, sitting, standing, and reaching. Practitioners may also sometimes work with the energy field surrounding the person. The goal of the work is the student's enhanced well-being and empowerment rather than physical healing per se.

OSTEOPATHIC MEDICINE Like M.D.s, osteopathic physicians provide comprehensive medical care, including preventive medicine, diagnosis, surgery, prescription medications, and hospital referrals. In diagnosis and treatment, they pay particular attention to the joints, bones, muscles, and nerves. They are specially trained in osteopathic manipulative treatment—using their hands to diagnose, treat, and prevent illness.

PAST-LIFE/REGRESSION THERAPIES Past-life therapy and regression therapy are based on the premise that many physical, mental, and emotional problems are rooted in the past—whether from childhood traumas or from experiences in previous lifetimes. The practitioner uses hypnosis (or altered states of consciousness) and relaxation techniques to access the source of these unresolved problems and helps clients to analyze, integrate, and release past traumas that are interfering with their current lives.

PATHWORK Pathwork, a personal-growth process incorporating spirituality and psychology, encourages the individual to face and transform his or her "dark side" or shadow with the goal of promoting integration, inner peace, and activation of the soul's greater consciousness. Through verbal dialogue, the practitioner assists the individual in removing physical, emotional, mental, and spiritual blocks often related to past traumas.

PHOENIX RISING YOGA THERAPY Phoenix rising is a form of yoga therapy designed to help clients achieve greater spiritual balance in their lives. A therapy session combines hands-on support in performing yoga postures with therapeutic dialogue techniques.

PHOSPHOTIDYLSERINE (PS) A type of fat found in all cells in the body but especially in brain cells. PS is found in small amounts in foods such as fish, soy products, and leafy green vegetables and is also available in supplement form. Some studies have linked PS supplementation by adults to improvement on memory tests.

PILATES METHOD The Pilates method is a full-body exercise system that emphasizes body alignment and correct breathing. With the help of an instructor, clients perform strength, flexibility, and range-of-motion exercises on specially designed equipment. The Pilates method may be performed by people of any age group or fitness level in order to improve their flexibility and range of motion. People in physical therapy may also use the method to aid in their recovery.

PLACEBO EFFECT An improvement in the condition of a sick person that occurs in response to treatment but cannot be considered due to the specific treatment used.

POLARITY THERAPY Polarity therapy asserts that balancing the flow of energy in the body is the underlying foundation of health. Practitioners use gentle touch and guidance in diet, exercise, and self-awareness to help clients balance their energy flow, thus supporting a return to health.

PREGNENOLONE A natural precursor to steroids that is converted by the body to hormones such as DHEA, testosterone, progesterone, and estrogen. Animal studies suggest that pregnenolone may help enhance cognitive function.

QI GONG Also referred to as chi-kung, this is an ancient Chinese exercise system that aims to stimulate and balance the flow of *qi* (*chi*), or vital energy, along the acupuncture meridians, or energy pathways. Qi Gong is used to reduce stress, improve blood circulation, enhance immune function, and treat a variety of health conditions.

REBIRTHING Also known as conscious-connected breathing (or by some practitioners as vivation), rebirthing is a technique in which the therapist guides clients through breathing exercises to help them reexperience past memories—including birth—and to let go of emotional tensions long stored in the body.

REFLEXOLOGY Reflexology is based on the idea that specific points on the feet and hands correspond with organs and tissues throughout the body. With fingers and thumbs, the practitioner applies pressure to these points to treat a wide range of stress-related illnesses and ailments.

REIKI Practitioners of this ancient Tibetan healing system use light hand placements to channel healing energies to the recipient. While practitioners may vary widely in technique and philosophy, reiki is commonly used to treat emotional and mental distress as well as chronic and acute physical problems, and to assist the recipient in achieving spiritual focus and clarity.

RELAXATION RESPONSE The relaxation response occurs through the meditative repetition of a word or short phrase—and the gentle return to this repetition whenever distracting thoughts occur—in order to trigger a series of physiological changes (slowed breathing, heart rate, blood pressure, etc.) that offer protection against stress. The relaxation response has been proven beneficial in treating stress-related conditions such as muscle-tension pains, insomnia, and hypertension.

ROBERT JAFFE ADVANCED HEALING ENERGY Developed by a physician, this healing approach uses "heart-centered awareness," clairvoyant perception, and a variety of energetic healing techniques to identify, understand, and transform the energy patterns that are believed to cause disease. Advanced healing energy is used to treat physical disease as well as emotional and spiritual disorders.

ROLFING This technique uses deep manipulation of the fascia (connective tissue) to restore the body's natural alignment, which may have become rigid through injury, emotional trauma, or inefficient movement habits. The process, developed by biochemist Ida P. Rolf, involves 10 sessions, each focusing on a different part of the body.

ROSEN METHOD Developed by former physical therapist Marion Rosen, the Rosen method combines gentle touch and verbal communication to evoke relaxation and self-awareness. Because the work can bring up buried feelings and memories, it is used as a tool for personal growth as well as pain relief.

RUBENFELD SYNERGY METHOD The Rubenfeld synergy method uses gentle touch, movement, verbal exchange, and imagination to access memories and emotions locked in the body. The approach, developed by healer Ilana Rubenfeld, integrates elements of the Alexander technique, the Feldenkrais method, gestalt therapy, and hypnotherapy. Because it combines bodywork and psychotherapy, The Rubenfeld synergy method may be used for specific physical or emotional problems or for personal growth.

SHEN THERAPY (the acronym stands for "specific human energy nexus") seeks to release deeply embedded painful emotions through the use of light hand placements. The practitioner applies his or her energy flow to the client's clothed body, thus seeking to "unblock" the client's energy flow. SHEN therapy is primarily used to treat some chronic pain syndromes, as well as physio-emotional disorders such as stress-related disorders (gastric problems and migraine headaches, for example) and general anxiety disorders (often associated with childhood sexual or physical abuse). SHEN therapy is also known as SHEN physio-emotional release therapy.

SHIATSU The most widely known form of acupressure, shiatsu has been used in Japan for more than 1,000 years to treat pain and illness and for general health maintenance. Using a series of techniques, practitioners apply rhythmic finger pressure at specific points on the body in order to stimulate *chi*, or vital energy.

SOMA NEUROMUSCULAR INTEGRATION This bodywork method seeks to improve posture, joint function, and body alignment through deep manipulation of the muscular and connective tissue. The 10-session process, which incorporates movement training, also seeks to promote greater access to the functioning of each brain hemisphere. People with conditions such as chronic back pain, arthritis, asthma, scoliosis, and headaches have sought relief through this method.

SPIRITUAL/SHAMANIC HEALING Practitioners of both spiritual healing and shamanic healing often regard themselves as conductors of healing energy or energy from the spiritual realm. Both may call upon spiritual "helpers" such as power animals (characteristic of the shaman), angels, inner teachers, the client's higher self, or other spiritual forces. Both forms of healing can be used as part of treatments for a range of emotional and physical illnesses.

STRUCTURAL INTEGRATION A systematic approach to relieving patterns of stress and impaired functioning, structural integration seeks to correct misalignments in the body created by gravity and physical and psychological trauma. As in Rolfing, in 10 sessions the practitioner uses hands, arms, and elbows to apply pressure to the fascia, or connective tissue, while the client participates through directed breathing.

TAI CHI/MARTIAL ARTS The martial arts are perhaps best known as means of self-defense, but they are also used to improve physical fitness and promote mental and spiritual development. The highly disciplined movements and forms are thought to unite body and mind and bring balance to an individual's life. "External" methods (such as karate and judo) stress endurance and muscular strength, while "internal" methods (such as tai chi and aikido) stress relaxation and control. Tai chi has been used as part of treatments for back problems, ulcers, and stress.

THERAPEUTIC TOUCH Co-developed by nursing professor Dolores Krieger and healer Dora Kunz, therapeutic touch is practiced by registered nurses and others to relieve pain and stress. The practitioner assesses where the person's energy field is weak or congested and then uses his or her hands to direct energy into the field to balance it.

TOUCH FOR HEALTH A self-help technique taught by instructors, touch for health is a system of balancing the body's energy by applying gentle pressure to contracted muscles and other points along the body. Regular balancing is used to improve overall health and strengthen resistance to common ailments and physical complaints.

TRAGER BODYWORK Developed by Milton Trager, M.D., this movement-education approach seeks to address the mental roots of muscle tension. By gently rocking, cradling, and moving the client's body, the practitioner encourages the client to see that physically restrictive patterns can be changed. Trager bodywork is meant to promote relaxation and increase mobility and mental clarity. It is used by athletes for performance enhancement, as well as by people with musculoskeletal and back problems.

TRIGGER POINT/MYOTHERAPY Practitioners of this technique apply pressure to specific points on the body to relieve tension. Trigger points are tender, congested spots in muscle tissue that may radiate pain to other areas. Though the technique is similar to shiatsu or acupressure, this therapy uses western anatomy and physiology as its basis.

VEGETARIANISM Vegetarians follow a meatless or mostly meatless diet. Vegans avoid all foods of animal origin, including meat, fish, poultry, eggs, and dairy products. Ovo-vegetarians eat a vegan diet plus eggs, lacto-vegetarians eat dairy products, and lacto-ovo-vegetarians eat both. Pollo-vegetarians eat chicken, and pesco-vegetarians eat fish.

VIBRATIONAL HEALING Practitioners of vibrational healing (also called vibrational medicine) use a variety of modalities that seek to promote healing by balancing the client's energy field. Such modalities may include homeopathy, flower essences, acupuncture, and energy-based bodywork practices such as therapeutic touch and polarity therapy.

VISUALIZATION A technique that uses the imagination to help patients cope with stress and encourage healing. Patients attempt to heal physical and emotional ailments by imagining positive images and desired outcomes to particular situations. Visualization with the help of a practitioner is known as guided imagery.

WATSU (WATER SHIATSU) Watsu, or water shiatsu, is a form of massage performed in chest-high body-temperature water. The practitioner guides the client through a series of dancelike movements while using Zen shiatsu techniques (stretches and finger pressure) in order to release blockages in the body's meridians, or energy pathways. Watsu is used to release tension and to treat a wide variety of physical and emotional problems.

YOGA Yoga is a general term for a range of mind/body exercise practices used to access consciousness and encourage physical and mental well-being. Some forms concentrate on achieving perfection in posture and alignment of the body; others aim at mental control to access higher consciousness. Between these two are forms of yoga that focus on the interrelationship of body, mind, and energy.

ZERO BALANCING Zero balancing is a method for aligning the body structure and body energy. Through touch akin to acupressure, the practitioner seeks to overcome imbalances in the body's "structure/energetic interface," which is said to exist beneath the level of conscious awareness. Zero balancing is often used for stress reduction.